## History of Medicine

It is sobering to realise that as recently as the year in which On the Origin of Species was published, learned opinion was that diseases such as typhus and cholera were spread by a 'miasma', and suggestions that doctors should wash their hands before examining patients were greeted with mockery by the profession. The Cambridge Library Collection reissues milestone publications in the history of Western medicine as well as studies of other medical traditions. Its coverage ranges from Galen on anatomical procedures to Florence Nightingale's common-sense advice to nurses, and includes early research into genetics and mental health, colonial reports on tropical diseases, documents on public health and military medicine, and publications on spa culture and medicinal plants.

## A Chemical and Medical Report of the Properties of the Mineral Waters

In medical terms, 'mineral water' was, in the early nineteenth century, any water that appeared to have an effect on human health. British physicians often prescribed mineral waters from particular locations – most commonly those at Bath – for a variety of illnesses. However, there was little available information on the chemical composition of these waters, and extant manuals were often inaccurate. This report by the physician Charles Scudamore (1779–1849) appeared in 1820, the first of its kind for decades. Having visited several well-known spas and wells, including Bath, Buxton and Cheltenham, Scudamore conducted a series of experiments on water samples: he reports using litmus, turmeric and violet papers to judge alkalinity levels; documents testing for various minerals using anything from soap to silver; and explains in detail the difference between hard and soft water. His report remains insightful reading in the history of medicine.

Cambridge University Press has long been a pioneer in the reissuing of out-of-print titles from its own backlist, producing digital reprints of books that are still sought after by scholars and students but could not be reprinted economically using traditional technology. The Cambridge Library Collection extends this activity to a wider range of books which are still of importance to researchers and professionals, either for the source material they contain, or as landmarks in the history of their academic discipline.

Drawing from the world-renowned collections in the Cambridge University Library and other partner libraries, and guided by the advice of experts in each subject area, Cambridge University Press is using state-of-the-art scanning machines in its own Printing House to capture the content of each book selected for inclusion. The files are processed to give a consistently clear, crisp image, and the books finished to the high quality standard for which the Press is recognised around the world. The latest print-on-demand technology ensures that the books will remain available indefinitely, and that orders for single or multiple copies can quickly be supplied.

The Cambridge Library Collection brings back to life books of enduring scholarly value (including out-of-copyright works originally issued by other publishers) across a wide range of disciplines in the humanities and social sciences and in science and technology.

# A Chemical and Medical Report of the Properties of the Mineral Waters

*Of Buxton, Matlock, Tunbridge Wells, Harrogate, Bath, Cheltenham, Leamington, Malvern, and the Isle of Wight*

CHARLES SCUDAMORE

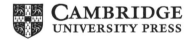

# CAMBRIDGE
## UNIVERSITY PRESS

University Printing House, Cambridge, CB2 8BS, United Kingdom

Published in the United States of America by Cambridge University Press, New York

Cambridge University Press is part of the University of Cambridge.
It furthers the University's mission by disseminating knowledge in the pursuit of
education, learning and research at the highest international levels of excellence.

www.cambridge.org
Information on this title: www.cambridge.org/9781108062022

© in this compilation Cambridge University Press 2013

This edition first published 1820
This digitally printed version 2013

ISBN 978-1-108-06202-2 Paperback

A

# CHEMICAL AND MEDICAL

# REPORT

OF

## THE PROPERTIES

OF THE

# *MINERAL WATERS*

OF

| | |
|---|---|
| BUXTON, | CHELTENHAM, |
| MATLOCK, | LEAMINGTON, |
| TUNBRIDGE WELLS, | MALVERN, |
| HARROGATE, | AND THE |
| BATH, | ISLE OF WIGHT. |

---

## By CHARLES SCUDAMORE, M.D.

*Member of the Royal College of Physicians,*
*Of the Medical and Chirurgical Society of London, &c. &c.*

---

## London:

PRINTED FOR THE AUTHOR,

By Joseph Mallett, 59, Wardour Street, Soho;

AND SOLD BY LONGMAN, HURST, REES, ORME, AND BROWN,

PATERNOSTER ROW.

1820.

MY LORD,

As, in the extensive series which this volume includes, the waters of Buxton first engaged my attention, I have placed it at the head of the list.

The antiquity of the Buxton springs is indeed of very early date; but so entirely have all the arrangements, made for the comfort and advantage of the invalid of every rank, sprung from your Grace's Family; and so manifestly do they continue to flourish under your patronage and direction; that it is with peculiar satisfaction I embrace the high honour allowed me, of presenting to your Grace the whole of the following Treatise.

With this sincere, though inadequate, testimony of respect, I have the honour to remain,

MY LORD,

Your Grace's most obedient,
and obliged humble Servant,

## CHARLES SCUDAMORE.

6, Wimpole Street,
Sept. 30, 1820.

# PREFACE.

HAVING the opportunity, in the Autumn of last year, of visiting several of the most remarkable watering places in this country, I became naturally inquisitive into the state of their mineral springs; and upon a slight examination of those which came first within my observation, I found reason to suspect the fidelity of the existing sources of authority respecting them. Books were defective in describing the number of the springs in many places, and more or less erroneous as to the chemical properties of most of the waters. I discovered the error into which I had been led by the confidence which I had placed in authors; and I resolved at least to gain some further instruction for myself. From one step I went on to another, and at length conceived an ardent desire to engage in an extensive inquiry into the subject, and present my results to the Profession and the Public, if they should appear to be sufficiently important in novelty and interest.

At Buxton, I was joined by Mr. Garden of
London, whose skill in operative chemistry is
well known. He brought all the necessary re-
quisites for making a complete analysis ; and we
afterwards proceeded to Harrogate. In every instance, all the preliminary experiments were
made at the springs ; but, except at these places
and Tunbridge Wells, the shortness of my stay
did not allow me the opportunity of examining
the gases in the usual method. In regard, however, to the saline waters of Cheltenham and
Leamington, and the more simple waters of
Malvern and Matlock, the determination of the
exact quantity of their carbonic acid, does not
appear to me by any means essential ; and the
proportions of sulphuretted hydrogen which some
of these waters contain, are, I think, made sufficiently evident for medical purposes. The
gaseous properties of the Bath waters are accurately stated by Mr. Phillips ; the analysis of the
aluminous chalybeate in the Isle of Wight is very
complete from the hands of Dr. Marcet ; and the
reprint of my former publication on the water of
Tunbridge Wells, embraces all that I could wish
to offer respecting it. The greater part of the
waters were wholly examined as to their solid
contents in London ; with all the care and repetition of experiments, which the importance of the
subject demanded.

To those acquainted with the difficult, and

almost endless details of chemical analysis, the
accomplishment of an investigation so extensive
will appear to be no trivial labour. Indeed,
I could not have engaged in it without some aid.
In addition, therefore, to the valuable assistance
which I received from Mr. Garden, I feel much
satisfaction in acknowledging my great obliga-
tions to my friend J. G. Children, Esq. whose
kind contributions will frequently appear in this
Work.

When the press every day teems with new
publications, it is a natural and fair inquiry, on
what grounds does an author offer himself to the
notice of the public ? My inducements on the
present occasion, I will further state.

The tepid springs of Buxton had not been
examined since the year 1784; the sulphuretted
and chalybeate springs of Harrogate, not since the
year 1794; and at Harrogate, a new and important spring had recently been discovered. I in-
clude also the report of several other new springs,
which have never been publicly noticed.

Modern chemistry has afforded improved
methods of analysis, and has led, consequently,
to new reasonings on the medicinal properties of
mineral waters.

I may be allowed, I hope, to add, without
impropriety, that I have engaged in this inquiry
with a mind wholly free from prejudice ;—free
also from the smallest partiality to any particular

place, or to the proprietor of any particular spring. My sole object has been to prepare a volume, which should contain a faithful statement of the chemical and medical qualities of the various waters of which I have treated. An annual excursion to some watering place has become so prevalent a fashion, that it is of importance to every medical practitioner to possess a manual, which shall safely guide his judgment in prescribing this class of remedies. The excellent Treatise, published by the late eminent Dr. Saunders, contained the best report on the subject which chemical analysis at that time of day enabled him to give ; but a sufficient interval has occurred, in conjunction with many changing circumstances, to render that work no longer an authority worthy of reliance.

I trust, therefore, that I have shewn the validity of my pretensions for appearing now in print. On the success with which I have executed the undertaking, the impartial critic must decide.

# CONTENTS.

————

# PRELIMINARY OBSERVATIONS.

———▶▶●◀◀———

In an extensive acceptation of the word, all waters, except rain water, might be named mineral; for, of necessity, they derive from the strata through which they pass, a certain degree of impregnation. But, in a medical sense, the term is limited to those waters, which, from their degree of impregnation, gaseous contents, or particular temperature, are found to produce some remarkable effect on the human constitution.

The first step in the examination of a mineral water, after having determined its specific gravity, is the application of certain tests or re-agents, with a view to form a general opinion of its composition.

For the information of the general reader, I shall prefix an explanation of such preliminary steps, and of the indications which belong to the respective re-agents that have been employed with the waters treated of in this volume.

*The specific gravity* of a water will alone

enable us to form a good conjecture as to the total quantity of solid matter which it may contain.

Kirwan, in his Treatise on Mineral Waters, gives the following formula for estimating the quantity of solid matter from the specific gravity, which, he states, will generally indicate the proportion within one or two per cent.

"Deduct, from the specific gravity of the water, the number 1000, and multiply the difference by 1·4; the product will represent the quantity of solid contents. It gives the weight of the salts in their most desiccated state, and consequently freed from their water of crystallization. The weight of fixed air must be also included.

Example.—Let the specific gravity of the mineral water be 1·079, and that of distilled water 1·000. Then $1079 - 1000 \times 1·4 = 110·6$, or, 100 parts of water of that sp. gr. should, according to Kirwan's rule, contain 110·6 parts of saline matter. He adds " that Brisson found a solution of two ounces of salt in 16 of water to have its specific gravity 1·079 : here 18 ounces of the solution held 2 of salt. Now as 18:2 :: 1000:111·1.

*Litmus paper* is employed to discover the presence of free acid in water, by which its blue colour is changed to red. This acid is usually the carbonic ; but a similar effect takes place from sulphuretted hydrogen. The redness thus

produced disappears after exposure to the air for
some time, or, is prevented by boiling the water
for a few minutes; and in this way the action
of these gases may be distinguished from that of
the other acids, which permanently redden litmus.

*Turmeric and violet papers* are delicate tests
for detecting uncombined or carbonated alkalies.
By these bodies the yellow colour of the former
is changed to a reddish brown, and the blue of
the latter to a green. A carbonated earth, as, for
example, carbonate of lime, has no effect on turmeric, but gives a green hue to the violet, even
when its proportion is very minute; such is the
great delicacy of this test.

There are other delicate tests for uncombined alkali, of which I may have occasion to
make mention.

*Tincture of galls,* when added to a water containing iron, produces a violet colour, or dark
purple, which, by standing, becomes more or less
black, according to the quantity of metal contained
in solution. If the change of colour be produced
previously to the water being boiled, but not
afterwards, it is a proof that the iron has been
held in solution by a volatile acid, as the carbonic. If, both before and after boiling, the
same change be produced, then we infer that the
iron is combined with a more fixed, or mineral
acid, as it is usually denominated.

*Prussiate of potash* is also a delicate test

B 2

for discovering iron when dissolved in a mineral water. The appearance which it presents with this metal, as the impregnation is weak or strong, varies from a pale greenish blue, to a dark Prussian blue colour.

*Lime water* is rendered turbid by waters which hold carbonic acid in solution. It does also occasion a precipitate with sulphates, and more especially when either sulphate or muriate of magnesia is present. If the precipitate which is produced by this test be soluble with effervescence in muriatic or nitric acid, it may be considered as carbonate of lime, and, consequently, that it has been occasioned by the carbonic acid of the water; but if its solution take place without effervescence, it has been produced by some of the other salts just mentioned

The same may be said if the water give a precipitate with lime water in its natural state, and fail to do this after boiling. In such cases, the precipitation is to be ascribed to the presence of carbonic acid alone; but should the water be sensibly affected by this agent both before and after being boiled, it may be considered that both carbonic acid and some of the salts just stated, are contained in the water. At least, the latter may with much certainty be expected.

*Nitrate of lead** is decomposed by sulphates

* It is to be understood that all the re-agents are to be employed in a liquid state.

and muriates : by the former salts, even though
their proportion be small ; but not by the latter,
unless they are present in considerable quantity.
This test also produces a black flaky precipitate,
if sulphuretted hydrogen be contained in the
water.

*The acetate of lead* is more usually employed
with a water suspected to contain sulphuretted
hydrogen. The colour of the precipitate produced by either of these re-agents, varies from
pale chocolate brown to deep shades of black,
according to the degree of the gaseous impregnation.

*Solution of soap* is decomposed, and produces
a flaky precipitate in any water which contains a
considerable proportion of any saline ingredient,
and especially by an earthy muriate, or a sulphate.

I may here observe, that the kinds of water
which are in domestic use, are commonly divided into *hard* and *soft* ; and that this distinction has been deduced from the difficulty or
facility with which the respective kind forms an
admixture with soap. If difficult, the inference
follows that much saline matter is contained.
The acid of the salt attracting the alkali of the
soap, leaves the oil detached, forming flakes or
curds in the water.

*Solution of barytes.*—The effects of this test
are, in some respects, similar to those of lime
water, in discovering the presence of carbonic

acid. It acts in the same manner, but is more delicate in discovering the presence of any earthy or alkaline sulphate, with which it forms a precipitate; and this precipitate (unlike that produced by lime water) is insoluble in nitric acid.

*Subcarbonate of soda* forms a precipitate with all the earthy muriates and sulphates, provided they exist in any considerable proportion.

*Muriate of lime* is decomposed by carbonated alkalies, if they be present in any notable quantity. The precipitate occasioned by a carbonated alkali, is soluble with effervescence in nitric or muriatic acid.

*Carbonate of ammonia, and phosphate of soda.*—These salts are chiefly employed in conjunction, for the purpose of discovering, in an unequivocal manner, the presence of magnesia. If a precipitate be produced by carbonate of ammonia when added in slight excess, the fluid is to be filtered; and, if then by the addition of phosphate of soda, it yield a further precipitate of a granular appearance, and adhering to the sides of the vessel, it may be considered that a magnesian salt exists in the water. The first precipitate is to be regarded as carbonate of lime; but if none take place from the carbonate of ammonia, the water is to be treated with the addition of phosphate of soda as just stated.

*Nitrate of silver* is a valuable and most delicate test for detecting the presence of muriatic acid, and all its compounds. A precipitate formed by any of these substances with nitrate of silver, is soluble in pure liquid ammonia.

*Liquid ammonia* does not decompose salts of lime; but with magnesian salts, a light white flocculent precipitate is produced.

*Oxalate of ammonia* is affected chiefly by salts of lime; but not (or at least not immediately) by those of magnesia. It is a most delicate test for discovering very minute quantities of lime in every state of combination. It produces a dense white precipitate.

*Muriate and nitrate of barytes* are excellent re-agents for the discovery of sulphuric acid, and all its compounds. They form, with the sulphuric acid of the salt, a dense precipitate of sulphate of barytes, which is insoluble in nitric acid. Of these tests, the muriate is the most delicate.

I proceed now to my general report of the waters, and commence with those of Buxton.

# BUXTON.

———⬥———

BUXTON, during many centuries famed for its medicinal springs, distant from London 159 miles, is a considerable village in the north-west part of the county of Derby, bordering upon Cheshire, from which it is separated by a chain of high mountains, intersected by deep ravines. The whole of this angle of Derbyshire constitutes what is called the Peak hundred, a wild mountainous district, thinly inhabited, and presenting a rude character of country. The following may be offered as a brief geological description.

It is in a valley surrounded by hills. Those in the immediate neighbourhood are calcareous, and belong to that class called, in this country, mountain limestone. It is a very ancient formation of rock, enclosing numerous fossil remains of enchrinites, madrepores, &c.; and is also well known here by the name of Derbyshire limestone. It is older than the coal formation which is placed upon it. Some of the hills in the neighbourhood, as Mam Tor, are composed of a sandstone called the mill-stone grit, which is by some considered as one of the beds of the coal series. The mountain limestone is remarkable for containing many very large caverns, the origin of which is uncertain, but which appear to

have been occasioned, or at least widened, by
subterraneous waters. In the immediate neighbourhood of Buxton, Pool's Hole is the chief;
but, a few miles distant, the Peak Cavern, and
the Speedwell Mine, are of greater magnitude,
and are particularly entitled to admiration. Dr.
Short, in his History of Mineral Waters, remarks,
that Buxton has long been celebrated for its warm
springs, and that they appear to have enjoyed
considerable reputation in the cure of various
diseases, for a longer period without interrup-
tion, than almost any mineral water in the kingdom. As early as the year 1572, a Treatise was
written on the virtues of this spring, by a Dr.
Jones, of Derby; and it appears at that time to
have been a place of great resort from all the
neighbouring counties. Several remains of Roman antiquity have also been discovered at, or
near, this spot; which makes it probable that
this fountain was not unknown to that people.

The water, of which I am about to give the
chemical and medical description, rises very freely
by numerous fissures through the limestone,
as may be distinctly seen in the large public bath
when it has been nearly emptied. The well of
St. Anne, appropriated for drinking, was many
years ago removed, for the sake of convenience,
several yards from its former situation. The
water is conducted from the spring head through

an artificial sandstone channel\*: it falls into a large marble basin (called the well), which is enclosed in a handsome stone building, conveniently constructed for the protection of the invalid; open to the air in front, and secured from intrusion, after the regular hours of resort, by an iron gate.

In its passage from the spring it loses five degrees of temperature ; being, at the head of the large bath, 82°, but in the basin, 77°†. It also loses a considerable portion of free azotic gas.

### CHEMICAL HISTORY.

The water is perfectly transparent, and free from air bubbles. It is destitute of odour, and has no other taste than that of common spring water heated to the same temperature. It does not affect either litmus or turmeric paper. The temperature in the well is 77° Fahr. As the

---

\* Dr. Pearson mentions that the diameter of this artificial semi-cylindrical channel is about four inches. The rate of supply of the water is a gallon in a minute.

† The same author remarks, p. 155, vol. i. that the temperature of St. Anne's well is 81° to 81°¼. I estimated the temperature of the water as it flowed immediately from the pipe, and found it exactly 77°.

water falls from the pipe into the basin, large bubbles appear, which, upon examination, were found to be occasioned entirely by the mechanical action of the water; atmospherical air becoming entangled, chiefly, during its fall. The specific gravity of the water at 60°, is 1·0006; but immediately from the spring, at 77°, is 999.

## Effect of Re-agents.

Pure ammonia produces an immediate slight opalescence, and, after a short time, a light flocculent precipitate.

Oxalate of ammonia immediately renders the water milky, and soon a dense precipitate appears.

Lime water, and a solution of pure barytes, render the water slightly milky. The lime water has no apparent effect on the boiled water, and the barytic solution only a slight effect.

Solution of subcarbonate of soda immediately produces a slight opalescence.

Solution of carbonate of ammonia, a similar appearance.

Muriate of barytes, a slight cloud.

Nitrate of silver, a precipitate more dense.

Solution of soap, an opalescence, but no immediate flakes.

Nitrate of lead, an immediate dense cloud.

Muriate of lime, no change.

Phosphate of soda produces an immediate

slightly milky appearance ; and, with the addition
of carbonate of ammonia, a minute granular
precipitate.

Tincture of galls, no change.

The action of these re-agents leads to the
conclusion, that this water contains muriatic and
sulphuric salts with bases of lime and magnesia,
in small proportions.

### ANALYSIS OF THE WATER.

*Of the gaseous contents.* — Twenty-one and a
half cubic inches of water from St. Anne's Well,
were introduced into a glass flask furnished with
a bent glass tube, its extremity terminating under
a jar filled with mercury, standing in a pneumatic
apparatus.　The water was made to boil gently
for about fifteen minutes; during which time a
quantity of gas was collected, amounting to ·9
of a cubic inch.　By treatment with lime water,
it was reduced to ·76 ; and the residuary gas,
after deducting ·33 of a cubic inch for the volume
of atmospheric air contained in the tube and neck
of the flask at the commencement of the process,
was found to consist entirely of azote ; since it
was neither itself combustible, nor capable of
supporting combustion.　It amounted to ·43 of
a cubic inch.

*Of the solid ingredients.*—(A.) A wine gallon
of the water was evaporated in a glazed earthen

vessel to dryness. The saline mass, dried at the temperature of 212°*, weighed fifteen grains.

(B.) The soluble salts were taken up by digesting the mass in cold distilled water, and the remaining insoluble matter, dried at 212°, weighed 10·9 grains.

(C.) The solution in distilled water was evaporated to dryness, and the dry mass digested in alcohol of the specific gravity ·815, with a view to separate the earthy muriates, if any existed in the water. The alcoholic solution, when evaporated to dryness, afforded a saline mass, which deliquesced in a considerable degree by free exposure to the atmosphere.

(D.) The deliquescent saline mass obtained in the last process, was dissolved in distilled water, and decomposed at a boiling heat by a solution of subcarbonate of soda.

(E.) The precipitate thus procured, was treated with dilute sulphuric acid, and a solution was obtained, which, by spontaneous evaporation,

---

* This appears to be the most suitable temperature for the drying of precipitates. It is very important in the analysis of mineral waters, that uniformity of temperature should be observed in this particular. From inattention to it, we have occasion to see that chemists of character have given widely different results in analyses of the same waters. It is however to be observed, that in Spring a mineral water will be found much more diluted than in Autumn, by the admixture of communicating springs; and hence certainly some explanation presents itself of the fact in question.

yielded distinct crystals of sulphate of magnesia. These crystals were dissolved in water; and the solution, on being decomposed by subcarbonate of soda, gave a precipitate, which, after ignition on a piece of platina foil, weighed ·2 of a grain; equal to ·7 of muriate of magnesia.

(F.) The liquid of process (d.) from which the magnesia was separated, was saturated with nitric acid, and a solution of nitrate of silver was dropped in so long as any precipitate continued to be produced. A quantity of muriate of silver was thus obtained, rather more than equivalent to the proportion of muriatic acid requisite to neutralize the magnesia obtained in the last process, and hence it must be referred to a portion of muriate of soda, which had been taken up by the alcohol.

(G.) The saline residue left after the action of alcohol in process (c.) was dissolved in distilled water, and the solution divided into two equal parts.

(H.) One of the portions was concentrated by evaporation, and decomposed by a boiling solution of subcarbonate of soda. A minute quantity of precipitate was obtained, which by treatment with sulphuric acid yielded ·30 of sulphate of lime.

(I.) The other portion of the aqueous solution was treated by a solution of nitrate of silver, with which it yielded a precipitate of muriate of silver, amounting to 2·25 grs. equivalent to 1·05 of muriate of soda.

(J.) The 10·9 grs. of insoluble matter left in process (b.) were digested in acetic acid, and the solution, when assayed by oxalate of ammonia and pure ammonia, appeared to consist entirely of acetate of lime. It was decomposed by a solution of subcarbonate of soda; and the precipitate, when dried, weighed 10.4 grs. The remaining half grain was found to be insoluble both in acid and alkaline menstrua. It was converted into charcoal by the action of heat, and therefore may be considered as entirely consisting of vegetable and extractive matter.

From this analysis, the composition of the water appears to be, in one gallon,

Of gaseous contents,

|  | Cubic Inch. |
|---|---|
| Carbonic acid........ | 1·50 |
| Azote............. | 4·64 |
|  | 6·14 |

Of solid contents,

|  | Grains. |
|---|---|
| Muriate of magnesia.. | ·58 |
| ———— soda...... | 2·40 |
| Sulphate of lime...... | ·60 |
| Carbonate of lime .... | 10·40 |
| Extractive matter, and a minute quantity of vegetable fibres...... | ·50 |
| (Loss)........ ... ... | ·52 |
|  | 15·00 |

Such, then, are the results of the direct method of analysis by evaporation ; but 1 must not omit to offer a statement of the composition of this water, according to the ingenious and original views of Dr. Murray.* The chemical reader will remember, that his theory requires us to consider that the saline principles of a water really exist in that state of combination which forms the most soluble salts ; and not in the condition of salts very little soluble as ordinary analysis represents, and which is to be explained by the re-action of the elements of acid and base, which takes place during the process of evaporation.

According therefore to this mode of estimation, the constituents of the water will appear to be as follows :

Grains.

Sulphate of soda......  ·63
Muriate of lime......  ·57
Muriate of soda ......  1·80
Muriate of magnesia ..  ·58
Carbonate of lime ....10·40
Extractive matter & loss 1·20
_____
15·00
_____

Dr. Pearson's analysis gave the following results. From a gallon of the water he procured

---

* Trans. R. S. Edin. vol. viii.

fifteen grains and three quarters of solid contents, consisting of

Grains.

Carbonate of lime...... $11\frac{1}{2}$

Sulphate of lime........ $2\frac{1}{2}$

Muriate of soda........ $1\frac{3}{4}$

———

$15\frac{3}{4}$

———

Dr. Pearson found that the proportion of carbonic acid, in the Buxton Water, did not exceed the half of what is found in many common springs. He had the merit of discovering the separate existence of azote in this water, a principle which had never been detected by any preceding chemist in any water. In the imperfect state of chemistry, thirty-six years ago, the nature of azote was unknown, and he described it, " as being a permanent vapour, composed probably of air and phlogiston." The present analysis gave about one-fifth more of azote in a gallon, than appears from Dr. Pearson's conclusions.

### MEDICAL HISTORY.

The properties of this water, as an internal remedy, have not been held in the same general high estimation as the baths, but yet their established reputation is considerable ; and the well of St. Anne is most commonly visited regularly

c

by the invalid, in conjunction with the plan of
bathing. It has been sometimes entertained,
even as a medical opinion, that the water can
scarcely act medicinally, otherwise than as tepid
water taken in the stomach, when empty, may be
considered to have a beneficial operation. This
conclusion has been drawn from the slight impregnation which the water possesses. A short
discussion on the question may not be uninteresting. Is the water medicinal from its minute
proportion of solid ingredients, and, in this respect,
its purity? Experience with some other mineral waters serves to shew that we ought not to
appreciate their power, merely in the ratio of
their impregnation. We consider that the water
of Bath derives a great part of its stimulating
power from the iron which it contains; and yet
its proportion, according to the analysis of
Phillips, does not exceed one-sixth of a grain
in the gallon.

In judging of the activity of any medicinal
ingredient in a water, we are to consider that it
exerts its influence under the most favourable
circumstances; and these chief advantages may
be thus stated. The substance is in a state of the
most minute division; its fluid vehicle is received into the stomach when free from food, so
that it acts readily upon the whole surface of this
sensible organ; and, lastly, it becomes quickly
absorbed into the circulation, not requiring,

like aliment, any stay in the stomach for the purpose of digestion.

The active material substances in the Buxton water are, according to the last view offered, sulphate of soda, muriate of lime, and muriate of magnesia ; but when we look at the very minute proportions, not a grain of either article in the gallon, and recollect that sea water, which, as an aperient, is taken without inconvenience, contains in the gallon 284 grains of muriate of magnesia, and rather more than 45 grains of muriate of lime, we are compelled to believe that the medicinal action of Buxton water must be referred to its purity, its temperature, and its gaseous impregnation with azote.

In every case, in coming to a final judgment of the medical character due to a mineral water, we must be very much governed by the records of the physician, and the report of the intelligent patient. Chemical analysis constitutes an important source of information, and is a material requisite in first conducting us to a scientific acquaintance with the water ; but subsequent experience and unprejudiced observation are necessary to give us practical knowledge, and a proper confidence in our remedy.

It is now incumbent on me to offer some observations, more precise, on the medicinal nature of Buxton water.

It certainly happens, that, simple as it appears in composition, it does prove inconveniently stimulating to some invalids of full habit and of the sanguineous temperament. They complain of flushing, head-ache, and slight giddiness; and are deterred by such symptoms from proceeding in the course of drinking it. Instances have come under my immediate observation, in which, the exciting power of the water has been proved in the gouty patient; symptoms of a paroxysm having occurred in a few days after its commencement, subsiding also upon its being discontinued, and with the assistance of aperient medicine. I intend this statement, however, only in illustration of my first remark; and by no means to deter the gouty patient from its use; who, on the contrary, will often derive much advantage from a course of the water, in common with others who suffer from derangement of the digestive organs.

As a general rule which will scarcely require any exception, it is expedient that one or two doses of suitable aperient medicines should be taken as a preliminary to the use of the water; and gouty patients ought not to begin a course of it, unless they are well prepared, and rendered free from every discoverable sign of an active state of the gouty diathesis.

The first dose of the water should be taken

about an hour before breakfast*. The medium quantity for the adult will be half-a-pint twice a day; and this portion should be drunk at twice, with the interval of a quarter of an hour, walking exercise being used, both in this interval and afterwards; or any other exercise, according to the capability and the convenience of the invalid. At twelve or one in the day, the same quantity of water should be taken upon the plan already stated. In the space of a week or ten days, the total quantity of water per diem may be increased to a pint and a half; but I am not aware that advantage is to be expected from proceeding beyond this quantity.

Such patients as find the water to be too exciting, notwithstanding that they have taken proper preparatory medicine, should make trial of it between breakfast and dinner, instead of drinking it before breakfast upon an empty stomach. Should it even then prove too stimulating, it might be tried with more chance of success, if previously allowed to remain in the open glass about a quarter of an hour, both to lose some of its temperature, and more particularly a portion of its gaseous matter. Should the water, however, thus treated fail to succeed, we must conclude that

---

* It is proper to drink the water after, and not before, bathing. The interval of an hour, or rather less, before breakfast will be sufficient.

there exists an inflammatory condition of the habit, requiring particular medical treatment; and
this having been premised, a better result from
the use of the water may be expected to follow.
The excitable patient, pursuing the plan of caution which I have just now stated, will most probably, by degrees, be enabled to drink the water
in its most active state.

The invalid of an opposite character of constitution, and daily accustomed to the free use of
vinous stimulus, will scarcely, if at all, be sensible of any immediate influence from the water;
and, looking to the simplicity of its composition,
may be disposed to regard it with great indifference. I have here, however, to add, that I have
seen instances in which the sanguineous temperament has not been favourable to the use of the
water, although the patient has been in the daily
habit of drinking a moderate quantity of wine
without suffering particular excitement. The
water taken before breakfast, in these instances,
produced head-ache, and flushing, and had the
same effect, in a less degree, in the middle of the
day. The individual possessing this constitution,
should be advised to exercise temperance and
careful regimen at the table, to forbear from the
use of much fluid at his meals, and to pay careful
attention to the due action of the bowels. If, even
with such observance, the water prove too exciting, the necessity will be manifest of employing

proper medical treatment, in order to reduce the inflammatory state of the habit. When the water agrees perfectly well, it sits pleasantly on the stomach, is refreshing, by degrees produces a sensible improvement of the appetite, assists the digestion ; and, thus amending the functions of the stomach, conduces to the general strength of the body, and consequent cheerfulness and comfort of mind. In concluding with a general medical character of the water, I may affirm that it proves very generally beneficial to the dyspeptic patient ; and that it is a valuable auxiliary to the use of the baths. In the condition of stomach which gout produces, and also in the state of constitution which is associated with chronic rheumatism, the internal use of the water has in many instances within my knowledge afforded decided benefit ; and, therefore, although it be less sensibly active in its properties than some of the other waters of which I treat in this little volume, it deserves, I am persuaded, to be regarded as considerably medicinal and useful.

Dr. Saunders remarks (Treatise on Mineral Waters) " that the inhabitants of the place employ the same water as common drink, and for all domestic uses which its hardness will admit of, and hence the invalid will probably take much more of the water than is prescribed, by its being used at table, and for culinary purposes." It is first to be observed, that, even if the water were taken from St. Anne's well for domestic use, it would so soon be altered with regard to its gaseous impregnation, that it would no longer be the same agent; and, in point of fact, the water used at the table was formerly taken from the two pumps near to St. Anne's well, each of which I found to furnish water at the temperature of 68°*; but of late, the pump behind the Angel Inn has been chiefly used. Upon examination of the water from this pump, I found that it had a considerable impregnation of iron; and hence I discovered the explanation of the unpleasant effect experienced by several individuals from drinking the water used at the tables of the hotels. They suffered from it head-ache and flushings. I have the satisfaction to add, that, by the recommendation and exertions of Dr. Drever, a water has recently been introduced into Buxton from a spring in the Manchester road. The specimen of the water, with which I was favoured by Dr. Drever, was remarkably pure, and free from all metallic impregnation.

---

* I was informed that one of these pumps furnished warm water, and the other cold; but, upon examination, I found that the temperature of each was 68°. It has always been stated, and indeed mentioned as one of the seven wonders of the Peak, that these contiguous pumps (within 12 inches of each other) furnished, the one warm water, and the other cold. Dr. Drever assures me of this fact, and that the cause of my finding the contrary was owing to an accidental communication between the springs.

# OF THE BATHS,

## *AND THE RULES OF BATHING.*

In addition to the large charity bath, which is used for the infirmary patients, there are three distinct baths for gentlemen, and two for ladies; besides which, there are excellent marble baths for the purpose of warm bathing; a vapour bath, and shower baths, most conveniently constructed, near to the general baths; and there is an excellent cold plunging bath at a short distance from the town.

The gentlemen's public bath measures in length 25 feet 4 inches; in width 17 feet 11 inches; in depth 4 feet 9½ inches.

The gentlemen's new bath measures in length 20 feet 11 inches; in width 10 feet 11 inches; in depth 4 feet 8½ inches.

The gentlemen's private bath measures in length 20 feet 6 inches; in width 6 feet 2 inches; in depth 4 feet 9 inches. The ladies' public bath measures in length 22 feet; in width 12 feet 8 inches; in depth 4 feet 5½ inches. The ladies' private bath measures in length 11 feet 6 inches; in width 4 feet 6 inches; in depth 4 feet 5¼ inches.

The baths are furnished with an excellent pumping apparatus, by means of which water is

projected with any degree of force upon particular parts of the body affected with disease ; and
there is a chair for the convenience of those infirm
invalids who are deprived of the use of their
limbs, with such machinery attached to it, that
the patient can be lowered into the water, and
raiséd, with great facility.

I must take notice of a deficiency of free ventilation in the apartments of the bath, which I
hope will in future be remedied.   The temperature of the  water will not be affected by having
the atmosphere of only moderate warmth, and
rendered free from oppressive steam by means of
careful ventilation ; while the patient will be more
comfortable in his sensations, and also be less
susceptible of injury from subsequent exposure
to the open air.*

The baths which are in regular use should be
emptied and refilled every day, and the utmost
cleanliness should be observed in the bath itself,
the apartments, and in all the arrangements ; such
attention serving not only to increase the comfort of the invalid, but also to render the bathing
itself more salubrious.   A thin stratum of steam
generally hovers over the baths, which is more
or less visible, accordingly as the temperature of
the apartment is more or less warm, and the air

* I will also venture to express a hope, that a better arrangement may be adopted in regard to dressing apartments.
At present this kind of accommodation is very deficient.

confined. Large and small air bubbles are constantly rising up through the water, which ex-
pand and burst as they arrive at the surface.
These bubbles are the most numerous in the
large bath, which is situated over the spring ; for
the smaller baths are supplied from the reservoir
of this spring on the gentlemen's side. The temperature of the public bath is 82° ; of the private
bath 82° ; of the new bath 81° ; it losing one degree of temperature in its longer course from the
reservoir. The largest bath can be emptied in
about ten minutes, and refilled in less than half
an hour. The smaller baths are emptied and
filled in a proportionably shorter time.

The large bath on the ladies' side, over the
spring, is 82°; but the private bath, which is supplied from the reservoir, is 81°, losing a degree
in its course.

The charity bath is 80° in its temperature.
Its size is 10 feet 8 inches, by 10 feet; the depth
4 feet 8 inches.

The cold bath is distant about a third of a
mile from the crescent. Its temperature in
November 1819 was 60°. Formerly this bath
was divided into two parts, the one for gentlemen, and the other for ladies; but they are now
laid into one. The bath therefore differs in
depth, being in one part 4 feet 9 inches, in the
other 3 feet 11 inches.

The specific gravity of the water of the reservoir* at its natural temperature, 82°, is 998·4, but at 60°, 1·0004.

The gas which rises in the form of bubbles through the public bath, is incapable of supporting combustion. A lighted taper immersed in it was instantly extinguished. With a portion of this gas, no change of volume was produced either by lime water or barytic water, and although mixed with an equal volume of atmospheric air, it almost instantly extinguished a lighted taper without the least explosion.

The composition of the water of the reservoir is similar to that of St. Anne's Well, as indeed must be expected, the waters being derived from the same spring. We have no reason to believe that the water of the well contains less of azotic gas in chemical solution, than that of the reservoir. The difference therefore will be in the temperature, as already stated, and in the circumstance of a considerable proportion of free azotic gas appearing in bubbles.

I am now to consider the medical use of the bath.

The invalid visiting Buxton may not have

---

* The experiments were made on the water of the reservoir on the gentlemen's side.

been prepared in the state of his constitution, so as to enter upon the use of the bath with the greatest advantage. In the instance of a plethoric habit, and more especially if there be marks of congestion in the vessels of the head, some loss of blood will be a necessary preliminary. If there be increased action in the general circulation, blood will be taken from the arm with more propriety; but when there is mere local fulness of vessels, not affecting the general circulation, cupping, or the use of leeches, will deserve a preference. Some suitable aperient medicine should be premised; and, obviously, an attention to the regulation of the bowels must afterwards be constantly observed. To this point I have already adverted, when speaking of the water of the well for internal use. I think it however necessary to remark, that mercurial medicine should be avoided during the immediate employment of the bath. The temperature of 82° is not sufficiently high to favour that action of the skin, which conduces to the safe and favourable action of mercurial alteratives.

The class of patients resorting to the Buxton bath comprise, for the most part, those who have suffered either from gout or rheumatism. But it is by no means equally proper for the gouty and the rheumatic invalid under circumstances apparently similar. I should forbid the use of the bath to a patient actually suffering the pains of chronic gout; and I should consider him to be requiring suitable medicines to remove such a diathesis, as an essential preliminary. The bathing will be a valuable remedy to relieve that debility of limbs, and of the whole constitution, which is a common sequel to chronic gout, and which seems to partake very much of the character of rheumatism. When gout, from the frequency and severity of its attacks, has not only debilitated the limbs in a serious degree, but has also weakened the constitution, so that the circulation is very languid, and the nervous system much depressed, it appears to me that a course of warm sea beathing, sea air, and friction, should precede the visit to Buxton; or, if circumstances do not allow this arrangement, the warm bath at Buxton may be the previous remedy, the temperature being gradually reduced to prepare the patient for that of 82°.

With respect to rheumatism, so long as it partakes of the acute species, the Buxton bath is not proper; and I am led to believe that patients have often been injured by thus prematurely using the bath. Even when there is local inflammatory action, not raising any general febrile irritation, as discoverable by the pulse, the immersion in the bath is seldom found to agree. But, flying general pains, with a natural state of the pulse, do not constitute an objection. It is in a rheumatic state of the constitution, unattended

with fever; when the various textures concerned
in muscular motion are so much weakened, that
the patient experiences lameness, stiffness, and
irregular pains, more particularly in damp
weather, before rain, and from a change of wind
to the east, that we see the happiest effects of the
Buxton bath. The distensions of the bursæ mucosæ, which form soft swellings near the large
joints, become relieved, and commonly receive a
cure, in a surprising degree of success, from the
influence of pumping on the affected parts, in
conjunction with the general bathing. This observation applies both to the effects of gout and
rheumatism. It will sometimes happen that the
patient (more particularly when rheumatism has
been the disease), whose infirmity is such that he is
conveyed with difficulty to the bath; whose dis-
abled state makes him require assistance at every
moment, and with difficulty is lifted into the
bathing chair to be let down into the water,—derives benefit so quickly, that in three or four days
he is capable of walking to the bath, and making
his own immersion; and the subsequent progress
of his recovery becomes wonderfully rapid.

The careful management of the bath is, in
several particulars, very important. Except in
certain instances of debility of constitution, it
is most advantageous to bathe before breakfast.
It is desirable that the patient plunge, instead of
stepping, into the bath. At first the stay in the

bath should in no case exceed two minutes ; and in many instances, one minute will be preferable. At the instant of the immersion, a slight sense of chilliness is experienced, but usually this is quickly succeeded by a moderate degree of warmth, sufficiently comfortable. The proof required that the bath perfectly agrees, is, that the patient derives from it an agreeable refreshment, a pleasant universal warmth, and a general increase of elasticity. The unfavourable effect is indicated by sensations of chilliness, lassitude, and indifference of appetite. Yet the bath must not be abandoned hastily, because its most agreeable effects do not immediately take place. The constitution may in a short time accommodate itself to the influence of the bath, although at first the result may seem rather unfavourable and doubtful. On this point however the patient should consult his medical adviser.

According to the nature of the case, and the individual constitution, the question must be determined whether walking or other exercise shall be taken immediately after the bath ; or, whether the patient shall rather refrain from exercise, or even take repose on the sofa.

Those who can use considerable exertion in the bath, and more especially in swimming, will not be so much restricted in the time of their stay, as others, whose infirmity permits only slight muscular action ; but in either case the time

should be gradually increased. For the debilitated patient (to speak by way of distinction), five
minutes may be stated as the full time ; for the
strong, ten or twelve ; and the increase of time at
each bathing, may be from half a minute to a
minute. When rheumatic painful sensations dis-
tress the patient, he should undress and dress
before a fire ; unless indeed the weather is quite
warm and dry.

Another point I wish to dwell upon, which I
think of particular importance, and this is, the
use of friction. I am convinced that the advantages of the Buxton bath would be most materially increased, if proper friction and *champooing*
were used immediately when the patient quits
the bath, or very shortly after. In this way, the
circulation of blood in the weak muscles is actively promoted, without the least fatigue to the
patient; and other good effects upon the infirm
limbs are by degrees produced. I may briefly
define the advantages of this practice to consist
in the influence which it may possess, to relieve
the parts from the effects of preceding effusion,
by exciting the absorbents to unload the cellular
membrane ; to assist in restoring the lost freedom
of motion in the tendons and ligaments ; to reno-
vate the capability of proper contraction and relaxation in the muscular fibres ; to improve the
circulation as above stated : and conduce to a

more perfect transmission of the nervous influence.

I shall hope to succeed in recommending this arrangement, as an addition to the general plan of Buxton bathing.

In regard to the theoretical consideration, whether a spacious bath filled with other water at the temperature of 82°, would afford equal advantages with the Buxton bath, it would be foreign to my present purpose to inquire. It is a question to be determined only by experience; and I am not acquainted with any bath of the same size and temperature in this country; so that the unrivalled claim of Buxton must, in this point of view, be fairly allowed. One obvious and important advantage derived from a spacious bath of the temperature of 82°, over a confined one at the same temperature, must be referred to the opportunity which it allows of free motion, and which materially assists the subsequent re-action of the circulation. It is indeed that happy medium of temperature between the warm and the cold bath, neither exciting by heat, nor depressing by cold, which enables it to act as a favourable tonic to the limbs, and to the general constitution. The uniformity of temperature in so large a body of water, could not be imitated in an artificial bath; and the possible influence which the azotic impregnation of the water may have upon the skin, is worthy to be considered.

On the present occasion I purposely avoid stating any of the cases of cure which have come under my observation, and within my knowledge. I have selected some striking instances of its success in another place*.

I should do injustice to my recommendation of Buxton, if I did not take notice of the remarkably bracing qualities of the air. Although, from its hilly situation, this district possesses a variable climate, yet, as the rain quickly disappears from the surface, the atmosphere is more remarkable for its dryness than its humidity. The invigorating power of Buxton air appears indeed to be generally acknowledged ; and I was informed by many invalids, that they became quickly sensible of its happy influence, receiving a remarkable improvement of appetite, of spirits, and of general energy.

The vicinity of Buxton is not devoid of interesting scenery, and affords the opportunity of some agreeable excursions, which will particularly gratify the lover of Nature in her rude attire. The most interesting objects are emphatically

---

* A Treatise on the Nature and Cure of Gout and Rheumatism, including general considerations on Morbid States of the Digestive Organs ; some Remarks on Regimen ; and Practical Observations on Gravel.

styled the Seven Wonders of the Peak ; but for all particulars of this kind, I must refer the reader to the information contained in the Buxton Guide.

The noble range of buildings called the Crescent, erected at the expence of the late Duke of Devonshire, furnishes, in its hotels, every elegant and comfortable accommodation ; and it may be added, that, under the fostering patronage of his Grace the present Duke, the several excellent arrangements at Buxton, established for the convenience and amusement of the invalid, or of the general visitor, as well as the institutions for charitable purposes, continue to prosper in the happiest manner.

## THE BUXTON CHALYBEATE.

In addition to the tepid springs which are peculiar to Buxton, there is also a chalybeate, which rises from a bed of shale, on the north side of the river, behind the George Inn.

It is a spring of weak impregnation, as the following statement will shew ; but it is a very pure water, and instances may occur in which its use will deserve recommendation. When it fails to produce so much effect on the constitution, as is required from a chalybeate medicine, it will be right to add, in suitable doses, and those gradually increased, the tinctura ferri am-

moniati.  For more extended observations on the
present subject, I refer the reader to my account
of the water of Tunbridge Wells ; and proceed
now to state some general chemical particulars
of the Buxton chalybeate.

The taste of the water is slightly and agreeably chalybeate.

The temperature is 54°.

The specific gravity is 1·0003.

### Action of Tests.

Tincture of galls in a few minutes produces
a violet hue.

Prussiate of potash, a light greenish blue.

After boiling, or after simple exposure for a
short time, no change of colour is occasioned by
these re-agents.

Nitrate of silver scarcely produces a change.

Nitrate of lead no immediate change ; but
soon a slight cloud appears.

Solution of soap scarcely disturbs the transparency of the water.

Lime water, no obvious change.

Muriate of barytes, a slight cloud.

Muriate of lime, no sensible change.

Pure ammonia causes a very slight brownish
precipitate, perceptible after standing.

Carbonate of ammonia, a similar effect.

Oxalate of ammonia, a slight cloud.

From the effect of these re-agents, we may infer that the iron in this water is held in solution by carbonic acid. From comparative experiments which I made on a former occasion with the different springs of Tunbridge Wells, and Tunbridge, I conclude that the proportion of iron in the water does not much exceed half a grain in a gallon.

It has only a small proportion of carbonic acid.

It contains a small proportion of the muriatic and sulphuric acids in a combined state.

It is a remarkably soft water.

# MATLOCK.

———

MATLOCK Bath is situated two miles from the village of Matlock ; 22 miles south-east of Buxton ; 17 from Derby ; and is distant from London 143 miles. Until its warm springs began to attract notice, about the year 1698, this sweet retreat was only occupied by the rude cottages of the miners. At that period the original bath was built, and a house also for the accommodation of visitors. Other buildings, as hotels and lodging houses, have since been erected ; and the place now affords every accommodation which can be desired.

Matlock Bath is placed in .a valley of the mountain limestone, close to the river Derwent, which at this spot is over-hung by mountain scenery of the highest order of picturesque beauty. The springs which flow into the Derwent, in many parts coat its borders with calcareous deposit called *tufa*, and which, with covering moss and vegetable matter, at length contribute to form a kind of embankment. Various substances are

thrown into these waters in their course to the
Derwent, in order that they may receive an in-
crustation from carbonate of lime, which the
water, on its exposure to the air, freely throws
down. Hence the term of the petrifying
wells.

Dr. Saunders quotes the following account
from Dr. Short's History of Mineral Waters :—
" A number of springs issue from the limestone
rock, all of them possessing the clearness and
purity that distinguish mountain streams which
rise from a clear rocky soil, but several of these
possess a temperature steadily above that of
natural waters in our climate. The cold and
tepid springs are singularly situated in this limestone hill. All the tepid waters arise from fifteen
to thirty yards above the level of the Derwent ;
whilst those both above and below are cold ; and
even the sources of the latter intermix with those
of a higher temperature." The supply of water
is very copious, and part is received into spacious
baths, used for medical purposes, and which
give the distinguishing appellation to this delightful spot.

### Of the Water at the Fountain.

The sensible properties of the water differ but little from common good spring water ; except, that its temperature, which is 68°, is in taste approaching to tepid.    It is beautifully clear, but does not sparkle much on being received fresh into the glass from the spring.  The fountain consists of a handsomely constructed vase*, of the Derbyshire marble; and its form and neatness, together with the transparency of the water, offer a pleasing invitation to the invalid to take a morning draught of this pure beverage.

The specific gravity of the water at 60° is 1·0003.   I had not an opportunity of making the examination immediately as it came from the spring.

### Action of Tests.

Litmus paper receives a reddish tinge, which disappears on drying.

---

* The pipe which conducts the water into the vase does not rise above half an inch from the bottom ; and when there is no water in it, the *jet d'eau* rises several feet ; but when the orifice is covered by a stratum of water, it only bubbles and flows over.

By the water in a very concentrated state, turmeric paper was not affected ; nor did it change paper stained with the flower of the wild hyacynth * ; a remarkably delicate test for alkali, and acting in the same manner as the violet.

Lime water renders the water slightly milky.

Solution of soap produces only a slight opalescence.

Nitrate of lead, a dense cloud.

Subcarbonate of soda, no change.

Muriate of lime, no change.

Carbonate of ammonia alone, no change ; but phosphate of soda being added, a slight cloud appears.

Nitrate of silver produces an immediate cloud.

Muriate of barytes, a dense cloud.

Oxalate of ammonia, a dense cloud.

Pure ammonia, no change.

Tincture of galls, no change.

From the effect produced by these re-agents, we are led to conclude that the water contains free carbonic acid, and some muriates and sulphates in minute proportion. From the further indications, the bases may be considered, as magnesia, lime, and probably soda.

When the water is concentrated by evaporation, it deposits carbonate of lime, and is then

---

* The hyacinthus non scriptus of Linnæus, and the scilla nutans of the Flora Britannica.

but very slightly affected by oxalate of ammonia. From comparative experiments made with precipitants, for the purpose of obtaining a nearer estimate of the relative proportions of the different salts, it appeared that carbonate of lime was the most considerable ingredient, and that the other salts, which are certainly in very minute quantity, were in about equal proportion. It is obvious that a water so slightly impregnated as this of Matlock, requires, for its complete analysis, that a very large quantity of it should be evaporated, and much time and labour bestowed in executing the processes. For all medical purposes, the present chemical view will, I trust, be found quite sufficient.

### MEDICAL HISTORY.

I have only a brief account to offer of the medical properties of the Matlock water, as an internal remedy. Dr. Saunders remarks, " that it may be employed in all those cases where a pure diluent drink is adviseable." It may truly be stated that the water can never fail to prove a wholesome beverage. It seems calculated to be really useful in dyspepsia, and in gravel. At the same time, I do not feel authorised to extol the water as a relief for any particular class of disorders. Its purity, its agreeable temperature, and its freshness, ensure to the invalid that, while it has the chance of being in some measure useful, it will not disagree.  The immediate impression on the stomach is more grateful than that occasioned by ordinary spring water ; is more tonic ; and when attention to regimen is joined with a course of it, much decided advantage may be expected.  This latter consideration must be allowed great weight, when applied to the case of the *bon-vivant.*  The adoption of a plan which is positively correct, and the avoiding of habits positively wrong, will be an important salutary change ; and, hence, the pure draught of Matlock water in exchange for the feverish cup of wine (I speak of excess), will every day conduce to the improvement of the stomach, and of the general health.

Half a pint of the water should be drunk an hour before breakfast, taking with it a small portion of biscuit.  A walk or ride should follow. The same draught should be taken at noon ; and again an hour before dinner ; exercise being duly used after each quantity.

The smallest measure of fluid which is convenient, should be used at meals ; for otherwise, it is probable, disadvantage will arise from distension.  The ordinary principles of medical management, as regards the regulation of the bowels, are, of course, to be observed.  Any kind of aperient medicine will be compatible with the waters ; but, as a general direction, I should advise the use of pills.

## OF THE BATHS.

At the two houses called the Old and New Baths, there is one large bath ; each about 22 feet in length, and 15 in width ; but near the *Museum*, adjoining the Fountain and New Walk, is a bath about 30 feet long and 18 wide. The natural temperature of the water in each bath is 68°. There are several hot baths, and a shower bath, so that a considerable gradation in a plan of bathing is conveniently obtained at Matlock. In speaking of a complete scale of bathing temperatures, I may mention the following series.— The hot bath of Bath ; the tepid bath of Buxton ; the bath of Matlock, which is just intermediate between Buxton and the sea ; the sea ; and, lastly, the cold bath.

The immersion in the Matlock bath at first produces a slight shock, but less than the cold bath, and it is soon followed by a re-action and an agreeable glow. Its use is very applicable to a weakened frame, when the constitution is not in that state of debility which prevents the necessary re-action from taking place.

It may be viewed as a promising remedy in certain states of muscular debility left by acute rheumatism ; but its temperature is rather too low to make it suitable for established chronic rheumatism ; and I should consider it for the most part, inapplicable for a gouty person ; allowing particular exceptions which should always be well considered.

In commencing the remedy, the bath should not be used more than each other day, and afterwards two mornings in succession, omitting the third. The invalid who is incapable of swimming, or using much other muscular exertion, should not remain in the bath more than one or two minutes ; and the more active patient should limit his stay to five or six minutes. It is always desirable to make a sudden immersion, falling forward. The time of day should be before breakfast, or in the middle of the day, accordingly as the strength of the patient will allow ; the very delicate invalid obviously waiting till noon ;—and it should precede the drinking of the water at the fountain.

The inhabitant of Derbyshire will find, as I am informed, a mild winter residence in the vale of Matlock bath, it being much sheltered on all sides from the cold winds. The traveller will be well rewarded for his labour in reaching this beautiful spot, where Nature, barren and rude in the surrounding country, has here assembled all the charms of scenery with a profusion of taste ; breaking on the view like enchantment, after the previous toils of a cheerless journey.

My limits will not allow me to expatiate further on these beauties, or to enter upon any description of the natural curiosities of the situation. Mr. Mawe's museum at Matlock bath is rich in a collection of the minerals and rocks which occur in the valley; and its excellent arrangement renders it an interesting and fertile source of instruction and amusement.

# TUNBRIDGE WELLS*.

—

In the year 1816, when residing at Tunbridge Wells for the season, I directed my attention to the qualities of its mineral water. Finding that twenty-three years had elapsed since its former examination by Dr. Babington, and an apprehension having subsequently arisen, that the water might possibly have suffered deterioration in consequence of the building of the baths near the spring, I was induced to submit it again to a chemical examination.

It is important to mention, that in this analysis I received the valuable assistance of my friend J. G. Children, Esq. a gentleman well known in science, and particularly distinguished by his celebrated experiments with the most magnificent galvanic battery, which has ever been constructed.

What I now offer, therefore, is almost a literal reprint of my former publication.

Tunbridge Wells is situated in that part of Kent called the Weald. The rocks in its neigh-

---

* I am induced to place the account of this water here, as I may have frequent occasion, in the course of the work, to make some allusion to its analysis.

bourhood are composed of a siliceous grit with a ferruginous cement, and belong to that series of beds which were deposited immediately before the chalk. In this part of the country, however, those beds are not covered by the chalk, which has been, most probably, carried off during one of those revolutions to which this planet has been subjected: but they may be traced passing under the chalk formation, along the bottom of the North Downs. This sandstone contains scarcely any fossil shells, but frequently iron in such abundance, that, before the discovery of the rich iron ore now procured from our coal works, this metal was procured in the Wealds of Kent and Sussex, where the remains of many ancient forges are yet to be seen. This ferruginous sandstone also alternates with thick beds of a tenacious clay, which forms a great part of the soil of this neighbourhood,

## OF THE SPRING.

The spring, which is now the only one in use, rises into a large marble basin. The water overflows through an aperture into a channel connected with the chalybeate cold bath, depositing in its progress a reddish brown precipitate.

### INTRODUCTORY EXPERIMENTS.

*Exp.* 1.—The temperature of the water as it

E

issues from the spring, is, in different seasons of the year, uniformly 50° Fahr. In the coldest winters it has not been known to freeze in the basin. On the 8th of February 1816, when the atmosphere was at 24°, the water in the basin was still at 50°. In the month of April, when I found some neighbouring springs yielding common water, and considered to be deep in their source, as low in temperature as 46° and 47°, this spring was still at 50°. In summer, the temperature of the water in the basin, near the surface, was raised a few degrees, in consequence of its free exposure to the sun's rays.

*Exp.* 2.—In examining the spring at different periods of the year, to ascertain its strength of supply, I derived the following results. In August 1815, it yielded, in a minute, one quart, two ounces, and five drachms. In the beginning of November, one quart. The summer had been unusually fine and dry. In October the season was wet. In the beginning of March 1816, the supply was increased to two gallons and a half in a minute. At the end of this month, the quantity was lessened to one gallon and seven pints. Much rain had fallen in the preceding months, but the winter had passed away with very little snow.

In the analysis of 1792, the specific gravity of the water is described " as exceeding that of distilled water, in the proportion of 713 to 712 ;" or as 1·0014 to 1·0000.

*Exp.* 3.—In several examinations of the water in the month of August, immediately fresh from the basin, and at its natural temperature 50°, I found its specific gravity compared with that of distilled water at 50°, as 1·0007.

### PHYSICAL PROPERTIES OF THE WATER.

The fresh water is perfectly transparent, and does not send forth air bubbles. It exhales a smell which is distinctly chalybeate. Its taste in this respect is strongly marked ; but is neither acidulous nor saline. It has an agreeable freshness, and is by no means unpalatable.

*Exp.* 4.—I put some small fish into the fresh water, and found that their respiration was immediately much distressed. One of them, a lively trout, was the most visibly affected, and died in three hours. The others, which were chubs, survived and recovered.

### SPONTANEOUS CHANGES OF THE WATER.

*Exp.* 5.—The water fresh from the spring, was exposed in a large glass vessel, in an apartment of the temperature of 68°. It quickly exhibited a few·air bubbles. In an hour a precipitation had begun, appearing in the form of a delicate white pellicle on the surface. This pellicle became thickened and shining in a few hours. In about six hours the water was faintly milky, and in twenty-four hours a slight brownish sediment had fallen to the bottom. In forty-eight hours the water became transparent; the pellicle was increased and beautifully iridescent. A brown precipitate was deposited, partly on the sides of the vessel, and partly appearing in diffused flakes. The water suffered no further visible change on longer exposure to the atmosphere.

*Exp.* 6.—Both the pellicle and the brown precipitate dissolved in muriatic acid, without the slightest effervesence.

*Exp.* 7.—The water contained in a corked vessel, received the before-mentioned spontaneous changes very slowly.

*Exp.* 8.—In a vial almost filled with the fresh water, and immediately sealed, no loss of transparency appeared during two days; but at the end of six days, the brown flakes were abundant. Both in this and the preceding experiment, the pellicle on the surface was very slight. A transparent glass bottle, in which the water has been frequently kept, though carefully washed, retains a strong iridescent stain.

*Exp.* 9.—Under the exhausted receiver of an excellent air pump, the spontaneous changes of the water took place much more slowly than when openly exposed.

## CHANGES PRODUCED IN THE WATER BY HEAT.

*Exp*. 10.—I immersed a thermometer in a flask containing the fresh water, and applied heat by means of a lamp.

At a temperature of 58°, the water did not suffer any apparent change.

At 60°, air bubbles became visible, and increased rapidly as the temperature advanced; but no other kind of change appeared until the water became heated to near 150°, its transparency till then not being affected.

At 160°, a faint milkiness was distinct.

The temperature increasing, air bubbles were still disengaged, and the whole liquor assumed a brown turbidness. Together with the brown flakes, which on the cooling of the water coalesced and subsided, minute vegetable fibres were very apparent.

### ACTION OF TESTS.

*Exp*. 11.—Tincture of galls dropped into the water, instantly produces a light purple hue, which in a few minutes becomes very deep. This, after an exposure to the air for two or three weeks, acquires almost the darkness and opacity of ink.

*Exp*. 12.—Prussiate of Potash in a few seconds strikes a light blue, which in a few minutes becomes azure, and, on longer standing, a fine Prussian blue is precipitated.

*Exp.* 13.—The water concentrated by boiling was not affected by either of the preceding reagents.

*Exp.* 14.—Tincture of litmus added to the fresh water, instantly produces a light pink red colour; which hue gradually escapes, and in a day or two changes to a lilac. Litmus paper is slightly reddened, but, on drying, returns to its natural blue.

*Exp.* 15.—The boiled water did not change the colour of the litmus tincture.

*Exp.* 16.—Syrup of violets, after a few minutes, causes a greenish tint, which gradually deepens, and at the end of twenty-four hours becomes a deep grass green. Violet paper is not instantly affected, but on drying assumes the green colour. No effect is produced on turmeric paper.

*Exp.* 17.—Oxalalate of ammonia produces no immediate change; but in two or three minutes, the transparency of the water is impaired, and it gradually becomes turbid.

*Exp.* 18.—Muriate of barytes produces an immediate slight cloudiness, with a few air bubbles, and a precipitate slowly subsides, which does not re-dissolve by nitric acid.

*Exp.* 19.—Nitrate of silver occasions blueish white streaks, and an abundant precipitate.

*Exp.* 20.—A solution of soap in alcohol, scarcely renders even the fresh water turbid.

*Exp.* 21.—Lime-water instantly produces a

faint milky hue; and a light brown turbidness immediately succeeds.

*Exp.* 22.—Nitro-muriate of gold, and nitrate of lead, occasion a slight disengagement of air-bubbles, without impairing the transparency of the water.

*Exp.* 23.—A few drops either of nitric, muriatic, or sulphuric acid, hasten the appearance of air bubbles; and this is so remarkable with the sulphuric, that it resembles effervescence.

*Exp.* 24.—A current of sulphuretted hydrogen gas being passed into the fresh water, no discolouration is produced; but if the experiment be made after it has been a short time exposed, it is rendered instantly black.

*Exp.* 25.—An infusion of tea, in a few minutes, strikes a purplish lilac.

*Exp.* 26.—A clear infusion of coffee is rendered of a blackish hue. With cocoa or chocolate, no change of colour appears to be produced.

### INFERENCES.

From the preceding experiments we derive the following conclusions;—but it should be remarked, that, with regard to the effect of re-agents, the indications can seldom be considered to possess more than general presumptive evidence.

1. It is certain that the spring rises from a great depth, *Exp.* 1.

2. That the state of the spring is considerably influenced by the seasons of summer and winter, *Exp.* 2.

3. The near approximation of specific gravity which the water possesses, to that of distilled water, is alone a proof of a small proportion of foreign ingredients, *Exp.* 3.

4. That the water contains iron, and probably in no very slight proportion, *Exp.* 10, 11, 12, 25.

5. That the iron is combined with carbonic acid, appears from the deposition of the reddish-brown precipitate in the basin, and along the channel through which the water flows, and from *Exp.* 5, 10, 13, 14, 24.

6. That the carbonic acid is the only solvent of the iron in this water. *Exp.* 13.

7. That the iron which exists in the water as a carbonate, falls down in its spontaneous separation, in the state of oxide, *Exp.* 6.

8. That free carbonic acid is contained in the water, *Exp.* 10, 14.

9. That the water contains a carbonated earth, is proved by the effect on the colour of violets, (*Exp.* 16); which substance, as was suggested by Dr. Saunders, requires separation from the iron with which it falls down, in order that the proportion of this metal in the water may be accurately estimated.

10. That a carbonated alkali is not present, is indicated by the colour of turmeric remaining unchanged, *Exp.* 16.

11. That lime is present, *Exp.* 17.

12. That the water contains combined sulphuric acid, *Exp.* 18.

13. That it contains a muriatic salt, *Exp.* 19.

14. That it is a soft water, is deducible from its low specific gravity, *Exp.* 3, and also from *Exp.* 20.

15. That the water is free from animal matter; and that the slight putrescence which it was found to acquire from confinement, when the pump was formerly in use, is referable to the vegetable matter which it contains, *Exp.* 22.

## MISCELLANEOUS EXPERIMENTS.

*Exp.* 27. To the boiled and filtered water, pure ammonia being added, after a few hours, a whitish flaky precipitate, very minute in quantity, is seen slowly subsiding; which, after remaining exposed two or three days, acquires a reddish-brown colour.

*Exp.* 28.—This precipitate being collected and dried, was fused with glass of borax, and the violet hue was produced;—being fused with pure nitre, a beautiful grass-green appeared. Prussiate of potash being added to a solution of the precipitate, a white precipitate instantly ensued. These results therefore were distinctive of the presence of *manganese*.

*Exp.* 29.—A portion of the ferruginous precipitate collected from the channel, and carefully
dried at a very moderate heat, was treated with
cold muriatic acid. It did not dissolve ; whence
it follows, that the iron thus separated from its
solvent, and exposed to the atmosphere, is in the
state of *peroxide.*

In the former analysis it is stated, that " the
whole ochre collected by the filter proved, when
dried, to be strongly *magnetic.*"

*Exp.* 30.—I found that no effect could be
produced by the magnet upon the ferruginous
precipitate, either after being dried by a moderate
heat, or being heated before the blowpipe ; but,
if heated with *wax,* it became strongly sensible.

### ANALYSIS OF THE SOLID INGREDIENTS.

Four gallons and 12 oz. (wine measure) of the
water were reduced by evaporation to three pints,
and the ferruginous precipitate was separated.
The remaining fluid was then evaporated to dryness. The solid matter, dried at 220°, was

|  | Grains. |
|---|---|
| Ferruginous | 11·9 |
| Saline | 19·6 |
|  | 31·5 |

|  | Grains. |
|---|---|
| Or, per gallon | 7·68 |

EXAMINATION OF THE SALINE MATTER.

A. 1.—The 19.6 grs. of saline matter were digested in 80 grs. of alcohol of the specific gravity of 805·72. After standing about eighteen hours, the spirituous solution was separated from the insoluble matter, and the latter washed with a little fresh spirit. The solution and washings were then evaporated, and the solid matter dried at 220°* weighed 2·85 grs. The solution was slightly tinged yellow, from a little vegetable matter taken up by the alcohol.

---

* The apparatus used for drying the precipitates, by means of heated air, consisted of a double cylindrical vessel of cast iron, with an intermediate space all around, and supported on legs, so as to receive a lamp under the bottom. A hole was perforated in the middle of the lid, to receive a thermometer; and the precipitate being placed on a stand conveniently adapted to the vessel, the heat of the enclosed air was easily regulated by the adjustment of the lamp. Double filters of equal weight were used, and the one dried with the precipitate as above stated, was again accurately weighed against the other. In the other analytical processes described in this work, we gave the preference to the method of decantation, employing small glass capsules, suffering the precipitates to subside, washing the matter with distilled water with the usual care, drying the precipitate in its capsule on sand heated to 212, and finally weighing the same, first with its precipitate, and afterwards freed from it with due care, thus estimating the weight.

2.—The 2·85 grains were decomposed by sulphuric acid, and evaporated, and the heat was raised towards the end, to expel the superfluous acid. The sulphate of magnesia was then carefully dissolved in a small quantity of cold water, and the solution separated from the sulphate of lime, which was again washed with a fresh portion of water. In this way a pretty complete separation of the two salts was effected, and the sulphate of magnesia being evaporated to dryness, and heated to 220°, weighed 1·6 grs. ; which was found by a separate experiment, made expressly for the purpose of comparison, to be equal to 1·22 of muriate of magnesia. This being deducted from 2·85 grs. leaves 1·63 gr. for the muriate of lime.

B. 1.—The saline matter, insoluble in alcohol, was dried at 220°, and weighed 16·75 grs. It was digested in 134 grs. of distilled water in the cold for several hours, and frequently stirred. The solution was separated, and the residuum washed in fresh portions of cold water. The washings and solution being evaporated to dryness, and heated to 220°, weighed 11·3 grs. and was common salt. On examination, however, it was found that some sulphate of lime was mixed with the muriate of soda. It was therefore redissolved, and muriate of barytes was dropped into the solution, as long as it produced any effect. When the precipitate had subsided, the clear liquid was separated, and the sulphate of barytes, which had formed, was well washed and dried at 220°.  It weighed 2·15 gr. =1·25 for the sulphate of lime ; which being deducted from 11·3 grs. leaves 10·05 of muriate of soda.

2.—The matter insoluble in cold water being dried at 220°, weighed 5·1 grs.  This was boiled with 5 oz. of distilled water, which dissolved the whole of the sulphate of lime, leaving only a small residuum, weighing ·6 of a gr.  This almost wholly dissolved with effervescence in diluted nitric acid, and the solution gave an abundant precipitate with oxalate of ammonia.  It was therefore carbonate of lime.  The portion not dissolved by the nitric acid, weighed ·02 of a gr. and was chiefly vegetable fibre, with some very minute particles of quartz sand.

### EXAMINATION OF THE FERRUGINOUS PRECIPITATE.

A. a. 1.—This precipitate (11·9 grs.), dissolved by the application of heat, in muriatic acid, with the exception of 1·8 gr. of a dark-coloured matter, which was found to consist of vegetable fibre, silica, and alumina.  The two last substances probably arose from some particles of dust accidentally blown into the basin from the walks, and mechanically suspended in the water.

a. 2.—The muriatic solution was diluted with more than a pint of distilled water, and pure ammonia, cautiously dropped in*, till the solution very slightly restored the blue colour of litmus paper, which had been reddened by vinegar. A copious precipitate of oxide of iron ensued. This was separated after standing some hours, and when dried at 220°, weighed 9·4 grs.

a. 3.—The clear liquid of the last process was evaporated to dryness, and the muriate of ammonia sublimed. When the volatile salt was quite driven off, and no more fumes arose on the application of a strong heat, a small portion of matter remained, weighing about half a grain, which consisted of carbonate of lime, and a slight trace of manganese.

The 9·4 grs. of oxide of iron being examined, by fusing a portion with pure potash, gave also indications of containing some manganese, but in quantity infinitely too minute to be estimated. The results of the foregoing analysis, therefore, appear to give,

---

* This method was adopted for the purpose of attempting the separation of the manganese from the iron, according to the ingenious method recommended by Mr. Hatchett, (Thomson's Annals, vol. ii. p. 343), which appears to me the best that has been proposed.

Of saline matter, 19·6 grs. consisting of,

A. 2. Muriate of magnesia............. 1·22
——————— lime................. 1·63
B. 1.  ——————— soda................10·05
B. 1 & 2. Sulphate of lime............. 5·75
    2. Insoluble.................... ·02
    Carbonate of lime............ ·58

                                 19·25

Of ferruginous precipitate, 11·9 grs. consisting of,

                                Grains.

A. a. 2. Oxide of iron............ 9·4
  a. 1. Insoluble............... 1·8
  A. 3. Carbonate of lime, &c..... ·5

                           11·7
                           19·25

                           30·95

                    19·6
                    11·9

     Total............ 31·5
     Ditto, by processes, 30.95

     Loss............ ·55

From these data, one gallon of the water appears to contain 7·68 grains of solid contents, in the following proportions.

Grains.

Muriate of soda.......... 2·46

———— lime.......... ·39

———— magnesia ....... ·29

Sulphate of lime .......... 1·41

Carbonate of lime.......... ·27

Oxide of iron............ 2·22

Traces of manganese, insoluble matter, (vegetable
fibre, silex, &c.)........ ·44

Loss in processes.......... ·13

———

7·68*

———

Or, stating the results according to the mode of computation of Dr. Murray, the following esti-mate will appear:

---

\* The whole contents of a wine gallon, according to the former Analysis of 1792, are stated as follows:

Grs.

Of Oxide of iron. ..................1·

— Muriate of soda..................0·5

— Muriated magnesia..............2·25

— Sulphate of lime................1·25

———

5

Cubic Inches.

Of Carbonic acid gas................10·6

— Azote...............................4·

— Atmospherical air..................1·4

———

16·

Grains.

Muriate of soda............1·25

Sulphate of soda...........1·47

Muriate of lime............1·54

———— of magnesia........ ·29

Carbonate of lime.......... ·27

Oxide of iron...............2·29

Traces of manganese, inso-

 luble matter............. ·44

Loss, &c.................. ·13

        7·68

## EXAMINATION OF THE GASEOUS CONTENTS OF THE WATER.

A flask which, with its ground-bent tube, contained exactly four ounces and a half of the fresh water, was completely filled by immersion in the basin. This water was gradually heated by means of a lamp, and the gas received over mercury. The boiling temperature was continued until no more gas came over.

The mean of three experiments, performed in this manner, the necessary estimates and corrections being made for barometrical pressure, assumed at the standard 30°, and for thermometrical temperature at 60°, gave, for the total quantity of gas, per gallon,

    Cubic inches. 13·3.

F

For the separation of the constituent gases, the usual methods * were adopted, and, as the mean of the several examinations, the following results were obtained:

Cubic Inch.

Carbonic acid, per gallon... 8·05
Oxygen................. ·50
Azote.................. 4·75
                        ────
                       13.30
                        ────

Or, stating the two last gases differently, according to the proportions † into which they enter to compose atmospherical air, it will be

Cubic Inches

Azote.................. 2·75
Atmospherical air......... 2·50

It has already been shewn, by *Exp.* 10, that the water may be heated to a very high temperature, without the smallest separation of the

---

* For the separation of the carbonic acid, lime water was the agent employed. The oxygen was separated by means of a solution of green sulphate of iron impregnated with nitrous gas. The residual gas was submitted to the power of the electric spark, and was proved by its negative properties to be azote.

† See these proportions stated in an excellent paper (the author Dr Prout), " On the Relation between the Specific Gravities of Gaseous Bodies and the Weight of their Atoms." Thomson's Annals, vol. vi. page 321.

iron.  Being further desirous, with a view to
medical considerations, to ascertain what influence should be produced on the proportion of
the carbonic acid gas of the water ; by the exact
temperature of the Bath water, 114°, being applied to it, the following examination was made.

The fresh water was heated by the lamp to
114°, and was then immediately transferred to
the flask already described, it, and the tube being
filled.  The remaining process was conducted
as in the former experiments with the fresh
water.

The mean of two experiments, the due estimates and corrections being made, gave for total
gas, per gallon,

Cubic inches,  9·14

The carbonic acid being separated in the usual
manner, afforded as the mean per gallon,

Cubic inches,  6·32

The following comparison, therefore, appears
from the whole results.

The mean of three experiments on the water
at its natural temperature, gave of

Cubic inches.

Carbonic acid gas, per gallon.........8·05
The mean of two experiments on the
   water previously heated to 114°.....6·32
                                        ————
Loss by heat.. 1·73

F 2

In reference to the variations in the quantity of supply which is yielded by the spring at different periods of the year, I have now to offer the results of comparative examinations of the proportion of iron in the water, at the following respective intervals.

Grains.

In August 1815, a dry summer preceding, and the supply of water in a minute being one quart, two oz. five drachms (*Exp.* 2.), of oxide of iron, per gallon........ 2·29

In the beginning of November 1815, much rain through October, and the supply in a minute being one quart (according to the analysis which has been detailed).... 2·29

On March 26, 1816, the supply in a minute being one gallon, seven pints.......... 1·63

It is hence shewn, that the strength of the spring, both in regard to its quantity of supply, and the degree of its chalybeate impregnation, is not connected with occasional changes of the season; but is to be referred to the gradual influence of the summer and winter upon the earth, which extends even to great depths*.

---

* Since this Analysis, I have made repeated examinations of the water. I found, in the very wet summer of 1816, the impregnation of the spring considerably weakened, although it endeavours to make up in quantity of supply in a given

EXAMINATION OF THE CHALYBEATE SPRING BE-
HIND THE SUSSEX HOTEL, WITH REFERENCE
TO ITS PROPORTION OF IRON.

Tincture of galls, dropped into this water, immediately produces a slight effect, but much weaker than on that of the Parade Spring. Making the comparison, I found, that in a few minutes, with the latter, the purple tint was very strong, but even at the expiration of half an hour, it was faint only in the former.

A similar distinction of result occurs from the prussiate of potash. No immediate effect is produced, and, after many minutes, only a very faint light sky-blue appears; while, in the Parade water, the change is instantaneous, and

---

time, what it wants in actual strength. Thus, in the beginning of November 1815, the spring yielded one quart in a minute. In October 1816, after a singularly wet season, the supply in a minute was no less than three gallons and a half. Its impregnation was proportionably weakened. I find that by comparing the effect of re-agents with the water, both as to the time and degree in which they act, with the results from the same re-agents, as I used at the time of making the analysis, I can form a very good estimate of the strength of the water as a chalybeate, at any particular time. This is always convenient, as pointing out whether or not some pharmaceutical preparation of steel should be joined with the use of the water.

in a very few minutes, a deep azure blue is produced.

One gallon of the water, procured in Sept.
1815, being evaporated, and the ferruginous
precipitate being separately obtained and dried at
the temperature of 220°, its weight was found to
be 1·1 gr.

ESTIMATE OF THE PROPORTION OF IRON IN A
CHALYBEATE SPRING NEAR THE TOWN OF TUN-
BRIDGE, CALLED THE TILE HOUSE SPRING.

One gallon of this water, procured in the beginning of November 1815, was evaporated, and
the ferruginous precipitate was separately obtained, and dried at 220°.   It weighed 1·77 gr.

In conclusion, I shall exhibit in one view a
comparison of all the results which have been
mentioned, with respect to the proportions of
iron.

Grains.

Parade Spring, Analysis of 1792, of oxide
    of iron...................per gallon, 1·
Ditto.........ditto.. Aug. and Nov. 1815.. 2·29
Ditto.........ditto.. March 26th, 1816.. 1·63
Spring behind the Sussex, ditto . . Sept. 1815. 1·1
Tile House Spring, near Tunbridge, ditto,
    Nov. 1815........................... 1·77

## ON THE MEDICINAL PROPERTIES OF THE
### WATER.

It has with truth been observed by Dr. Saunders, in his General Treatise, that "the most noted of the simple chalybeates in this country, is that of Tunbridge Wells\*."

It may with equal justice be added to this character of the water, that the mildness and salubrity of the air, joined with the remarkable beauty of scenery in the surrounding country, render Tunbridge Wells a situation of resort for the invalid at once valuable and delightful.

When it is considered how small a proportion of iron is contained in this water, in a quantity so large as a gallon of the fluid; and that the utmost portion thus taken by the patient falls so far short of the dose which is constantly administered in the preparations of pharmacy, it becomes a natural and interesting inquiry to determine, whether its powers as a medicine have all the pretensions which it claims; and how far the imagination may have contributed to the credit which it has acquired. I wish to meet this question fairly, and to apply the conclusions which may result from the discussion.

---

\* A Treatise on the Chemical History and Medical Powers of some of the most celebrated Mineral Waters, &c. 1800, p. 237.

Some persons, I know, when in perfect health, have made trial of the water ; and not finding from it any notable effect, have most unjustly undervalued its power, which ought not to be expected to act in any very marked manner, unless on the invalid.    An exception, however, presents itself to this observation, as I can assert, from experience, that all persons in full health cannot make free use of the water with equal impunity.    A plethoric habit, with vessels easily excited to strong action, might find it to be a very injurious stimulant.

It is admitted universally, both by medical and chemical writers, that the most active form in which iron can be administered as a medicine, is in the state of solution by carbonic acid.    I have already shewn, in *Exp.* 10, that in this water, the iron continues in perfect solution at a temperature a little beyond 140°, a heat full forty degrees higher than that of the human stomach. We may conclude, therefore, that in this state of perfect chemical activity, it exerts its agency in a very direct manner, over the whole of the surface of the stomach to which it is applied.    It is also probable, from the speedy and active diuretic power of the water, that the iron may partly find its way into the circulation, in its entire state of solution.

To the carbonic acid gas itself, a considerable and very useful influence may justly be assigned.

The small proportion of the solid ingredients in this water, which detain the carbonic acid in union, enables that agent to exert its effects more directly and actively upon the stomach ; and for the same reason, namely, the remarkable purity of the water, we may further explain why its virtues as a chalybeate are so remarkable as they are found, with relation to the actual quantity of iron.

The action which the azote may have on the stomach, is to be considered.

The manganese which is present may probably, as a tonic astringent, deserve some regard ; but from any particular speculations on this question, I shall forbear.

The saline ingredients, existing in the water in such minute proportions as I have stated, appear, with the probable exception of the muriate of lime, scarcely deserving of regard as medicinal substances.

It is obvious, therefore, that this water is distinguished by the remarkable purity in which it possesses a solution of iron, in carbonic acid gas ; and the investigation of its properties as a medicine, and the methods of its employment, I have now more distinctly to consider. It may be conceived that the most considerable, as well as the most immediate agency of the water is upon the stomach itself ; and that its impressions are secondarily communicated to the heart and arte-

ries through the medium of the brain and nerves
Hence the powers and good effects of the water
will be felt, according to the judicious preparation and fit condition of the stomach. This
important point of attention is too much over-
looked : and from this cause, from general erroneous management, and misapplication of the
remedy on the part of the patient, many of the
visitors of this Spring experience injury rather
than benefit. Some instances of this kind have
come under my own observation ; and many
have been related to me on the best authority.
It is equally true, on the contrary, that this water
judiciously employed, is a powerful and very successful remedy in many diseases.

A single dose of half a pint will contain, according to the Analysis which has been given, and
the statement made agreeably to Dr. Murray's
views, of solid ingredients, about $\frac{1}{100}$ of a gr. of
oxide of iron ; $\frac{8}{100}$ of a gr. of muriate of lime ;
$\frac{8}{100}$ of a gr. of muriate of magnesia; $\frac{8}{100}$ of a
gr. of muriate of soda , $\frac{8}{100}$ of a gr. of sulphate
of soda ; $\frac{8}{100}$ of a gr. of carbonate of lime, and a
minute portion of manganese ; and of gaseous
ingredients, half a cubic inch (or a quarter of an
oz. in bulk) of carbonic acid gas ; $\frac{7}{100}$ of a cubic
inch of azote, and about the same quantity of
atmospherical air.

On all occasions, on entering on the use of
this water, some aperient medicine should be

premised. If more than such simple treatment
be required, it constitutes a case in which further
medical consideration would be necessary. The
patient being favourably prepared, should take
the first dose of the water at seven or eight o'clock
in the morning ; the second at noon ; and the
third about three in the afternoon. A small portion of biscuit, with the dose of water before
breakfast, is to be recommended. In the middle
of the day this is optional. However small the
total quantity may be which is first employed, I
am induced to recommend this frequency of repetition, upon the same principles that we employ
any diffusible stimulant in successive portions,
where it is our object to render its effects permanent. The exact quantity to be taken daily,
must of course be varied, according to the several circumstances of the age and constitution of
the patient, and the nature of the disease ;—but
above all, according to the effects which it is
found to produce on the individual. The directions of the women in attendance (who are
named the *Dippers*) can only be of a general,
and obviously not of a medical nature ; but certainly, as far as relates to the *quantity*, they are
always on the side of security, supposing that
the case is not unfit for the employment of the
water.

It is very correct that every one should begin,
and continue, with a small quantity, for three or

four days ; after which, if it perfectly agree, the total daily amount should, I apprehend, be larger than is most commonly employed.

As a general statement, I would say that half a pint daily, is the extreme smallest quantity, and that two pints daily is the extreme largest amount, to found a just expectation of benefit; and further, in the way of general outline of direction, I conceive, that half a pint, a pint, a pint and a half, and two pints, should form the progressive ratio of the total daily quantity to be taken at the three intervals. As the patient arrives at the larger proportions, they may with advantage be subdivided, with the interval of a quarter, or half an hour, which should be occupied in exercise.

Those who consult their health in the best manner, should take exercise in the open air of the common, rather than in the sheltered parade, when the weather is favourable. I need not expatiate on the kind and degree of exercise, which must be entirely relative to the convenience and strength of the invalid.

An attentive regard to diet is strictly necessary. Tea at breakfast should be avoided, on account of the combination which its astringent principle forms with the iron in the water, as demonstrated in *Exp.* 25 ; and for the same reason, in a degree, the use of coffee also is not very correct. In the evening, however, either of

these refreshments may be taken without disadvantage, as the water will long since have quit-
ted the stomach.  Bread and milk, or cocoa, or
chocolate, may be taken at breakfast with propriety.  The hour of dining should not be later
than four or five*: and with this arrangement,
very slight refreshment only can be required in
the middle of the day    It is hardly necessary
to observe, that more than ordinary prudence
should be pursued in  the general diet, in order
to give the best opportunity of efficacy to the
water ; and, as a part of this plan, as little drink
as may be convenient should be taken at meals.
A want of caution in this particular, in addition
to other bad effects which it may produce, will
serve to weaken the stomach by over-disten-
sion.

    In many cases the coldness of the water will
have a salutary influence on the stomach.  It is
almost always judicious to allow it a fair trial at
its natural temperature, and with its complete
properties just fresh from the basin.  If, however, after a sufficient trial, it should sensibly
disagree, or should fail in producing the stimulating effects which are desired, its powers on the
system will, probably, be found much increased by

-------------------------------------------------

    * I would advise that not less than an hour should always
elapse between the taking of the water, and a meal.

giving to it an addition of temperature. The
failure in question will happen more especially
in those constitutions, where the circulation is
languid ; where the skin, and feet and hands, are
remarkably cold ; and where a great defect of
nervous energy is altogether apparent.   It is true
that by raising the heat of the water, rather less
of carbonic acid will be taken in the dose ; but
this loss will most probably be more than com-
pensated, by the increased stimulant power
which the chalybeate receives from heat.   This
observation will appear more consistent, when
we refer to the former position, that beyond 140°,
the iron does not escape from solution.   By the
*Exp.* p. 19, determining the loss of free carbonic
acid, which the water sustains from the heat of
114°, the practitioner is enabled to determine the
question for his patient, according to his own
judgment.   The agency of free carbonic acid
is certainly not to be disregarded ; and as being
the solvent of the chief active principle which
is administered in this water, its properties are
more especially important.   In some cases, I have
seen a very superior benefit produced from the
water, when taken cold from the basin, where I
should have feared that it would disagree ; while
in others, its active and useful operation has been
much assisted by heat.   Dr. Saunders, in his
general Treatise, commenting upon the activity
of the oxide of iron as a medicine, when held

in solution by carbonic acid, and assisted by
high temperature, as in the Bath water, in which
the greatest estimated proportion of iron is not
more than one-sixth* of a grain in a gallon,
remarks, " May we not therefore conclude, that
Bath water is indebted for its powers on the
human body (independently of those of mere
water at a high temperature) principally to the
circumstances of a chalybeate impregnation,
minute in itself, but much exalted in all its properties by a heat superior to that of most chalybeate springs ?" He adds, " that waters of the
description of Tunbridge Wells are best heated
by being put into a bottle well corked, and immersed in hot water."

It does not appear to me that any advantage
is gained by corking the bottle,—an operation
both tedious and liable to accident. It could not
be completely filled and then exposed to heat
with safety ; and when a free space is left in the
bottle, as necessarily must be, the withdrawing
of the cork allows the escape of all the free carbonic acid extricated by the increased temperature, as completely, as if its temporary confinement by the cork were neglected.

* Analysis of the Hot Springs at Bath, by Mr. Richard
Phillips.—Phil. Mag. vol. xxiv, p. 342. 1806.—This is the
latest Analysis, and doubtless the most accurate.

I recommend therefore as the most favourable mode, a thin glass flask, having a thermometer fixed in it.   The flask being dipped in
boiling water the necessary temperature is soon
communicated, and then instantly the water is to
be poured out for drinking.   No difficulty occurs
in executing this little plan.   If increase of temperature be really a medical object, as I affirm it
to be, it is important, both that the degree should
be adapted to the exact direction in the particular case, and also that it should be constantly
uniform; an advantage not to be insured in any
other way, than as I have now stated.

On the first employment of the water, either
cold or warm, some inconvenient sensations very
commonly arise, such as flushing of the face,
slight fulness of the head with drowsiness, and
an uneasy distension of the stomach with more
or less of flatulence.   In general these effects
are not of importance, either in degree or
duration; and are much to be prevented by previous attention to the stomach and bowels.   If,
notwithstanding this care, and the correct observance of general rules, the symptoms above-men-
tioned continue, the necessary inference is, either
that sufficient preparation has not yet been
made, or that the remedy is not suited to the
case.   Dr. Saunders expresses himself in the
following words: " The simple chalybeate produces no action on the bowels.   When these are

foul and loaded with sordes, the water often purges pretty briskly at first, but this operation ceases when the intestines are restored to their natural state."

I do not hesitate to affirm, that, in the occurrence of this faulty state of the bowels, the use of the water should not be begun; or, if taking place afterwards, that its continuance should be suspended, until suitable medicine has produced its proper effects. I may mention the following symptoms as certain indications of the necessity of some preparatory treatment;—a furred tongue, with heartburn, and occasional nausea; unnatural discharges from the bowels; and a turbid state of the morning urine, which, in a faulty state of the digestive organs, usually deposits, more or less copiously, a reddish or pink sediment, or one that is crystallized and commonly denominated gravel. As a general statement, it may be added, that the employment of this water is improper in a very plethoric state of the circulation, and especially when this is connected with any degree of inflammatory action. Also, when there is an inflammatory determination to any particular organ, or even when local congestion exists without inflammation. In cases of simple debility of the constitution, the water promises to produce its happiest effects. The proofs of its immediately agreeing with the patient, are, increased appetite and spirits; and

these auspicious symptoms are followed by a
gradual improvement in the general energy and
strength.  I was informed by many delicate dyspeptic patients, that they received a very sensible support from the water, so as often not
to feel the necessity of the ordinary recruit of
*luncheon* in the middle of the day.  Active exercise taken immediately after the water, produces with most persons a degree of general glow
of warmth, occasioned by the increased circulation, which may be a consequence very much
of a re-action succeeding to the impressions made
on the stomach by the *coldness* of the water.
The increased action of the kidnies is also a very
favourable indication of the salutary action of the
water ; and this effect is much promoted by
an adherence to the proper rules of diet and
exercise.

To speak again of the importance of immediate exercise, in the praise of which too much
cannot be said, it helps the water to sit lightly
on the stomach, to quicken its absorption, and,
in a word, to promote powerfully all its good
effects.

The bowels usually become constipated, and
require the assistance of medicine.  It appears
to me preferable for the most part, not to join
purgative medicines in mixture with the water,
lest the stomach be nauseated, but to give it at
bed-time in the form of pills.  Those containing

aloetic compound (as for example, the pulvis aloes compositus formed with the decoctum, or the pilul. al. c̄ myrrh.), I have found to be the most beneficial. In some instances, it may be found adviseable to add 20 or 30 grains of sulphate of magnesia to the water, the salt being previously dissolved ; and if taken with each dose of the chalybeate in such proportion, its effects may be secured, without the nausea that would arise from an occasional and larger quantity. I must repeat, however, that the conciliation of the stomach to the water itself, should seldom be hazarded by the addition of any nauseous combination. Also, the admission of the water into the circulating system, which is probably a consideration of importance, would be much opposed by any purgative admixture. This practice therefore appears to me correct, only in some cases of unfavourably astringent action of the water, together with a sensibly heating effect on the system.

The propriety of employing warm or cold bathing, in co-operation with the chalybeate, must be entirely relative to the individual case, and cannot form a part of a general outline of instructions. Dr. Saunders observes on this point, " It is frequently of eminent service to employ the warm bath occasionally ; and the propriety of this practice, strongly recommended by Hoffman, is amply proved by daily experience."

I cannot presume to offer an abstract of all the diseases, in which the water might probably be found a remedy ; but a few remarks, partly deduced from my own experience, and in part collected from authors, may not be unacceptable.

In dyspepsia, depending on debility of stomach, and accompanied with general languor and nervousness, a course of the water is remarkably restorative ; and it deserves a similar recommendation, in the debility which is more or less consequent to an active plan of treatment for the removal of bilious complaint.

In uterine debility, its tonic powers are very successful, both in improving the general functions of the organ, in lessening painful irritation and general irritability, and in restraining that inordinate action of the vessels which depends chiefly on their want of tone. Dr. Saunders, in reference to this point, and to the different forms of local debility thus connected, forcibly points out, that as they are " a very frequent cause of abortion or barrenness, these mineral springs have often been the means of removing such unpleasant circumstances."

In chlorosis, as might be expected, the water is eminently useful ; but from the languor of the system which so often accompanies this form of complaint, its employment requires much auxiliary management. It is here principally that its powers will often be much assisted by giving to it the Bath temperature of 114°; by joining the occasional use of the warm bath, employed so as not to produce its relaxing effects ; by acting on the bowels with aloetic pills ; and by enforcing a strict observance of the rules of diet and exercise ; of which last point of attention, the patient in these cases is generally too unmindful. It sometimes happens that in this complaint, a feverish irritation exists, accompanied with cough and pain of the side ; and certainly such symptoms demand removal, before the water can be entered upon with prudence.

As a remedy for that kind of cutaneous complaint which is connected with weakness of stomach, and which is usually of the scaly species, this water, by its tonic powers, promises to be useful. *Dr. Willan* concludes the mention\* of Tunbridge Wells water, amongst others, " as having been at all times particularly commended for their utility in the lepra, scaly tetter, and other cutaneous affections." He observes also†, " Chalybeate medicines are perhaps occasionally useful by removing states of the constitution, with which the scaly tetter seems to be connected." It is I

---

\* On Cutaneous Diseases, p. 111.　　† *Ibid.* 182,

think just to add my opinion, that the sulphuretted water of Harrogate, or even the saline waters of Cheltenham and Leamington, possess a greater efficacy in cutaneous diseases, than this simple carbonated chalybeate ; although where superior convenience for its employment does occur, it may deserve considerable confidence.

In scrophula, *the sea*, in its different modes of employment, has a much higher claim to our choice than a chalybeate water : yet, after a long trial of its powers, a change may on many occasions be usefully made, to the mild invigorating air of Tunbridge Wells; when the water also may be employed with great propriety, and with a prospect of much benefit. I am informed by a medical friend, of one very satisfactory example of the kind, in which, taken internally, and also applied externally to an ulcerated surface, it was useful.

As a stimulating diluent and diuretic, in addition to its tonic influence on the stomach, it bids fair, in conjunction with other treatment, to be useful in gravel, of which disease, an unhealthy condition of the digestive functions is the foundation. I have had some convincing proofs of its beneficial influence, under these circumstances. At the same time, the action of the bowels, and the state of the secretions should receive due attention. The acid matter which

continually forms in the primæ viæ in this disorder, should be neutralized by appropriate medicines.

The employment of the water for young children, is a much more questionable consideration
than for adults. From the observations which I
have attentively made, I am induced to draw a
*general* conclusion, that under six years of age
especially, it is not a favourable remedy. The
diseases of very young children are for the most
part of a nature to require a distinct attention to
the bowels ; to the progress of dentition ; and a
judicious arrangement of diet, exercise, and sleep,
with cold or tepid ablution, or bathing ; and do
not, so far as I have seen, come within the useful
influence of a chalybeate water.

In respect to the necessary duration of a course
of the water, it may in general terms be observed,
that a shorter period than three weeks scarcely
justifies the expectation of any material advantage ; and that a longer one than two months, or
at the utmost three, is not required, to produce
all the good effects of which it is capable ; so that
its employment has been fairly and judiciously
managed.

When after considerable trial, the water, although it may have agreed perfectly, yet has appeared deficient in power, I have been induced
to recommend an additional dose of steel from

the *Materia Medica.* Two or three grains of sulphate* of iron, formed into pills with five or ten grains of extract of bark or gentian, taken with each dose of the water, I can mention from experience to be very useful; and I may add another preparation, the tincture of ammoniated iron, in doses of twenty, thirty, or forty drops, mixed with the mineral water, as being a very successful auxiliary.

It remains for future experience to determine and record, to what extent more complicated cu-

---

* It appears to me that in the medicinal exhibition of iron, it is most commonly desirable to choose those preparations which have the greatest solubility, and which may accordingly be esteemed the most active. The rust of iron (Rubigo ferri, Pharm. 1787) does not afford the least effervescent action with muriatic acid, and may be considered a red oxide, very insoluble, and little capable of being acted upon by the stomach. The ferri subcarbonas of the present Pharmacopœia has a weak action on the addition of the acid, and may be viewed as a carbonated oxide. The precipitate which subsides from a mixture of a solution of sulphate of iron, and of carbonate of potash, exhibits a strong effervescence with the acid. Hence it may be stated as a conjecture, that so long as the iron remains in the state of black oxide, it retains more in proportion of carbonic acid, and parts with it, as it approaches to the state of red oxide. If a pharmaceutical preparation therefore of a carbonate of iron, on which the stomach may act with least difficulty, be attempted, Griffith's mixture (mistura ferri composita), used when recently prepared, claims our preference.

rative intentions may be effected, by joining the general or specific operation of other medicines, to the given range of action belonging to this carbonated chalybeate.

In conclusion of my present subject, I may observe, that the most favourable period of the year for the visit of the invalid to this fountain of health, is from May to November ; both because this season affords the best opportunity of enjoying the very material adjuncts of regular exercise, of early rising, and of the full influence of the air ; and because it gives the important advantage of drinking the water in its highest state of impregnation.

# HARROGATE.

THE villages of High and Low Harrogate are situated in an agreeable country, in the centre of the county of York, about three miles distant from the town of Knaresborough, sixteen from Leeds, twenty from York, and 211 from London. The whole of the neighbouring district abounds with mineral springs of various qualities, but principally sulphuretted and chalybeate; and Harrogate in particular has long enjoyed a high reputation by possessing valuable springs of both these kinds. Formerly the chalybeate water was the only one employed internally, whilst the sulphuretted was confined to external use. For many years past, however, the latter has enjoyed a large share of confidence as an internal medicine.

Several sulphuretted springs are met with, in the state of open wells, on the boggy soil, at a short distance above Low Harrogate, but they are less impregnated with the gas than the old sulphur well, as it is familiarly called. On the same level with this well, and not far distant, there are some springs of a similar character, but differing in strength. One of these is called the Crescent; and there are now three pumps belonging to the Crown Inn, each supplying a strong sulphuretted water.

The bog may be stated to consist of the remains of decayed vegetable matter, forming a black fetid half fluid mass, in many places four or five feet in thickness, which every where rests on a bed of clay and gravel. From hence the water appears to pass under ground through strata of shale; and having undergone a natural filtration in its passage, it rises perfectly transparent to the surface.

The mode in which the formation of sulphuretted hydrogen gas takes places, is a problem in the internal chemistry of the earth, which I cannot hope to solve. There are coal pits in the neighbourhood of Harrogate, and the probability may be suggested that the gas may be produced in the coal strata, as we know that it is formed during the making of coal gas. Water thus impregnated may afterwards traverse beds of salt, and then rise to the surface of the earth. Dr. Garnett supposes that the gas may be formed from the decomposition of pyrites, or sulphuret of iron, He also suggests, as a probable explanation, that the decomposition of vegetable matter furnishes hydrogen gas, and that this gas acts as a solvent to the sulphur. It does not happen that all bogs produce sulphuretted hydrogen gas. Might we not expect its more frequent occurrence, if the explanation could be referred to the decomposition of vegetable matter?

The Old Sulphur Well is almost the only one

of this description now resorted to as a drinking water, and the various additional springs are in full requisition for the use of the baths. The supply of this well is very abundant, and proves sufficient for the demand of the fullest season; allowing also of the exportation of a large quantity, in bottles, to distant parts of the kingdom. I commence my account with this water.

### OLD SULPHUR WELL*.

This water, when first taken up, appears perfectly transparent. It sends forth a few air bubbles. It has a very strong sulphureous and fetid smell, which has been compared to that of a damp rusty gun barrel. To the taste it is very saline, and disagreeable from its strong impregnation with sulphuretted hydrogen gas, for which flavour I know no comparison. It is however a remarkable instance of the power of habit in reconciling the palate to the most nauseous taste, that persons in general very soon can drink this water without disgust. It loses its transparency when exposed for about two hours to the air; at first acquiring rather a green hue, and after longer standing, by transmitted light, a slight reddish colour. It

---

* The water rises into a capacious stone basin, defended from the immediate falling of rain by a dome raised on pillars; a rude edifice, and very much demanding improvement, both for the purpose of more neatness and ornament, and greater security from weather.

gradually loses its sulphuretted taste, and then
has the flavour of a strong solution of common
salt. We found by experiment that the sulphuretted hydrogen gas undergoes decomposition
by exposure. The oxygen of the atmosphere
unites with the hydrogen, and the sulphur is precipitated in a state of minute division, the precipitate being of a light ash colour. Hence the
turbid appearance of the water. It is, however
extremely worthy of observation, that this water,
bottled at the spring, and immediately corked
and sealed, retains its gas and all its virtues for a
long time. I have examined bottles which have
been kept several months, and the water appeared to possess its gaseous impregnation unim-
paired.

The temperature of the water is 54°.

Dr. Garnett states the specific gravity of the
water as 1·0064. I found it, in different examinations at the spring, to be at its natural temperature 1·0103, but at 60°* 1·0101.

### Action of Tests.

Litmus paper was slightly reddened, but this
tinge disappeared on drying.

Lime water produced a slight cloud.

---

* I may here observe, that in taking the specific gravity
of all the waters, I used a bottle holding accurately 1000
grains of distilled water at 60°, and employed a balance which
was quite sensible to the 10th of a grain.

Acetate of lead, a copious dense precipitate, of a deep blackish brown colour. With the boiled water it produces a white precipitate.

Pure barytes, a light brown precipitate.

Pure ammonia, a dense precipitate, of a light brown colour.

Subcarbonate of soda, a similar effect.

Muriate of barytes, a slight cloud.

Oxalate of ammonia, a dense precipitate.

Nitrate of silver, a copious brown precipitate, with a shining pellicle on the surface.

Tincture of galls does not immediately disturb the transparency of the water, but soon a beautiful iridescent pellicle appears on the surface, the body of the water not being discoloured.

From these effects we may presume that the water contains muriatic and sulphuric acids, united to lime and magnesia, with a strong impregnation of sulphuretted hydrogen gas.

## ANALYSIS OF THE WATER.

*Of the gaseous contents.*—A. Sixteen cubic inches of the water were made to boil for about fifteen minutes in a glass flask connected with a Woulf's apparatus, into which a solution of acetate of lead, with excess of acid, had previously been introduced. In this manner a quantity, of sulphuret of lead was obtained, which, when edulcorated and dried, weighed 2·4 grs. This quantity may be stated as representative of ·951 of a cubic inch of sulphuretted hydrogen gas.

B. To an equal portion of water, as was employed in the last experiment, a quantity of acidulated solution of acetate of lead was added, and the gaseous product made to pass into a Woulf's apparatus, substituting for the acetate of lead in the bottles, a quantity of lime water. ·7 of a grain of carbonate of lime was deposited, representing ·66 of a cubic inch of carbonic acid gas.

C. The gaseous substances * contained in sixteen inches of the water, were collected in a graduated jar previously filled with water. The jar with its contents was suffered to remain inverted for many hours, during which time it was occasionally agitated with a view to facilitate the solution of such portion of the gaseous matter as might be soluble in water. There remained ·6 of a cubic inch of gas, which water did not appear to be capable of absorbing; and which, when exposed to the action of a solution of iron impregnated with nitrous gas, did not undergo any material diminution.

D. A portion of the residuary gas obtained in the preceding process, when mixed with oxygen gas in the proportion of one of the latter to two

---

* The corrections for pressure and temperature, as described at p. 65, were duly made.

of the former, and fired by the electric spark in a detonating tube over mercury, was diminished from ·30 to ·22 of a cubic inch, the total bulk of the mixture before explosion being ·30 of a cubic inch. Lime water thrown up into the tube became sensibly turbid, and the volume of gas was further diminished ·05. The residuary gas possessed the characters of pure azote.

Hence it would appear that the portion of gas insoluble in water consists of carburetted hydrogen, and of azote, in nearly equal volumes.

I may here mention that the gas which we collected from the open wells on the bog, which rises up in bubbles through the water, on being ignited in a large jar, burnt with a lambent blue flame ; but a taper immersed in a narrow jar containing this gas was instantly extinguished.

*Of the solid contents.*—A. A wine pint, or twenty-eight cubic inches of the water, slowly evaporated, yielded **106** grains of solid residue, dried at the usual temperature of **212°**.

B. This product was digested in alcohol for several days, and a solution of part of the saline contents was obtained. This evaporated to dryness gave a quantity of solid matter, which, by exposure to air, deliquesced considerably, and became nearly all dissolved. The deliquesced mass was dissolved completely in distilled water ; and the solution decomposed at a boiling heat by the addition of subcarbonate of soda. The precipitate thus obtained was treated by dilute sulphuric acid, and a quantity of sulphate of lime and sulphate of magnesia was produced, equivalent to 3·5 grs. of muriate of magnesia, and to 4 grs. of muriate of lime.

The fluid from which the earths were separated by subcarbonate of soda, was neutralized by nitric acid, and then decomposed by nitrate of silver. A quantity of muriate of silver was obtained, equivalent to 3 grs. of muriate of soda, deduction being made for the proportion of muriatic acid necessary for the constitution of the two earthy muriates, mentioned in the preceding section. The saline residue insoluble in alcohol was digested in distilled water, and the matter insoluble in this menstruum, amounting to 3 grs. was put aside for further examination. The watery solution was divided into two equal portions. The one portion was decomposed by a solution of subcarbonate of soda, and a precipitate of carbonate of lime was obtained, which, when dried, weighed ·2 of a grain.

The other portion of watery solution was treated in succession by nitrate of barytes, and by nitrate of silver. Precipitates were obtained of sulphate of barytes, and muriate of silver, equivalent to ·3 of a grain of sulphate of lime, and 46 grs. of muriate of soda.

The substance insoluble in water was acted

H

upon by acetic acid assisted by a gentle heat. A partial solution was effected ; which, by the addition of a carbonated alkali, gave a precipitate amounting to 1·9 gr. This precipitate, upon further examination, proved to be composed of 1·5 gr. of carbonate of lime, and ·4 of a gr. of carbonate of magnesia.

The residue insoluble in acetic acid was boiled in a solution of bi-carbonate of potash, and a further quantity of carbonate of lime was obtained, corresponding to ·4 of a gr. of sulphate of lime.

A minute portion of matter remained, which resisted the action of both acids, and alkalies ; and, from being almost entirely combustible, appeared to be extractive matter.

From this, the direct mode of analysis, the composition of the water appears to be in one gallon,

Of gaseous contents,

|  | Cubic inches. |
|---|---|
| Sulphuretted hydrogen | 13·716 |
| Carbonic acid | 9·529 |
| Azote and carburetted hydrogen | 5·800 |

These last gases appeared to be in about equal proportions.

———

29·045

Of solid contents,

|  | Grains. |
|---|---|
| Muriate of soda............. | 760 |
| ———— lime............. | 32 |
| ———— magnesia......... | 28 |
| Sulphate of lime............. | 8 |
| Carbonate of lime........... | 12 |
| ———— magnesia....... | 3·2 |
| (Loss)................. | 4·8 |
|  | 848 |

The composition of the water, if stated according to Dr. Murray's method of computation, will be as follows:

|  | Grains. |
|---|---|
| Muriate of soda.......... | 730·72 |
| ———— lime.......... | 55·10 |
| ———— magnesia...... | 32·35 |
| Sulphate of soda.......... | 8·32 |
| Carbonate of soda........ | 16·71 |
| (Loss)................ | 4·80 |
|  | 848·00 |

Dr. Garnett, in his analysis (the second edition of which bears the date of 1794), obtained the following results from a gallon,

Of gaseous contents,

|  | Cubic inches. |
|---|---|
| Sulphuretted hydrogen........ | 19 |
| Carbonic acid.............. | 8 |
| Azote..................... | 7 |
|  | 34 |

Of solid contents,

|                              | Grains. |
| ---------------------------- | ------- |
| Muriate of soda............. | 615·5   |
| ———— lime............ | 13      |
| ———— magnesia......... | 91      |
| Sulphate of lime............ | 00      |
| ———— magnesia........ | 10.5    |
| Carbonate of lime........... | 18·5    |
| ———— magnesia....... | 5·5     |

754

The difference of result between the present analysis and that by Dr. Garnett, does not allow of easy explanation. A different mode of operating, the particular season of the year at which the analysis is made*, and accidental variations in the water itself, are circumstances which are all to be considered. The period which has elapsed since Dr. Garnett's analysis, has brought about new views in chemistry; and, consequently, different estimates may have been formed as to the relative constitution of the salts. We do not obtain any sulphate of magnesia; but by Dr. Murray's mode of computation, we have almost an equivalent quantity of sulphate of soda. Dr. Garnett has not taken any notice of the presence of carburetted hydrogen in the water.

---

* The present analysis was made towards the end of September 1819.

## MEDICAL HISTORY.

THE water now under consideration unquestionably claims great medical regard, it being an agent of decided power and efficacy ; and, when its complicated gaseous composition is considered, it may be pronounced to be incapable of imitation by art.   It appears to have been in use nearly two hundred years, and its reputation, I believe, never has been higher than at the present moment.

It is important that the patient, on his arrival at Harrogate, should use some treatment preparatory to the drinking of the water.   One of a sanguineous temperament, and most certainly if labouring under plethora, should lose a few ounces of blood, which may be taken from the arm or by cupping, as circumstances shall indicate.   The gaseous properties of the water are considerably stimulating, and, from the neglect of this precaution of moderately reducing the circulation in certain constitutions, it is apt to occasion some heat and unfavourable excitement.

As a general rule, it will be expedient to administer a mercurial cathartic, consisting of a gentle dose of calomel and the compound extract of colocynth, in conjunction with the usual draught of senna and sulphate of magnesia.   In

any marked case of congestion in the circulation of the vena portarum, with a large abdomen,
and a sluggish state of bowels depending either
on the deficient and defective quality of the bile,
or upon the failure of its due excretion, it becomes important to pursue a course of the pilula
hydrargyri and the above extract combined, every
other night, upon an alterative plan.  Or, if any
circumstances in the constitution of the patient
forbid even this mild and guarded use of mercurial preparation, some suitable purgative pill
will be the proper auxiliary.  This water, it will
be seen from the analysis, contains but a small
proportion of the active aperient salt; and, with
many persons, fails to afford sufficient excitement to the bowels, so that some aid is abso-
lutely required.  This aid is in general more
usefully given by joining the use of a stimulating purgative pill, rather than by adding either
the sulphate of soda or magnesia to the water,
unless some particular circumstances in the case
suggest the propriety of doing this.  In many instances, also, it is our wish that the water should
act more decidedly as an alterative, and not pass
off rapidly by the bowels.

The patient should rise early, and repair to
the well to drink the water at the fountain head.
The advantages of this proceeding are obvious.
The medium dose may be stated to be three
quarters of a pint taken at two draughts; the

first quantity being half-a-pint. Some exercise, more or less active, according to the powers of the individual, should be used in the interval between the doses, which may be from twenty to thirty minutes. According to the age and constitution of the patient, and particular circumstances of the case, the doses now stated are to be exceeded or lessened. I conceive that the management of taking the water, must entirely depend upon the nature of the case for which it is administered; and the consequent kind of effect which is desired to be produced. If taken with a view that it may act quickly and decidedly as an aperient, auxiliary means, as just stated, being used if necessary, the whole quantity should be drunk before breakfast; but if, on the contrary, it be used more moderately as an aperient, and also as an alterative, the total quantity should be taken at twice; the first and larger portion before breakfast, the second and smaller in the middle of the day.

It is found useful by way of conciliating the palate, to eat a small portion of spiced gingerbread, or of brown bread at the time of drinking the water. The action of the morning doses is best promoted by the use of black tea for breakfast. It may happen now and then, but I should believe but very rarely, that the stomach does not receive the water so well in its natural state of coldness. Under such circumstances, it may be a little warmed by the addition of a small quantity of boiling water; but its gaseous properties are more perfect at its original temperature.

A full course of the water may be stated to require from four to six weeks, observing, during this period, an occasional interval of a few days. It is satisfactory to mention, that the Harrogate water confers a great share of permanent benefit; carrying on its good effects long after, upon the patient who has suffered from habitual torpor of bowels; and this, it must be allowed, is a result of great moment. I have before stated that this water bears removal and long keeping without any material diminution of even its gaseous properties; and, hence, the use of it may be continued, or resumed after an interval, when the patient has returned home.

The application of sulphur is so familiarly associated as a remedy for the diseases of the skin, that Harrogate has usually numbered among its visitors, a very considerable proportion of those who suffer from some form of cutaneous complaint. Its use, however, is every year becoming more extended towards other disorders; and it is found to be an active and important agent in exciting the action of the liver, and thus bringing about more regularity of function in the whole alimentary canal. In this description of visceral torpor, its employment in conjunction with the pilula hydrarg. and colocynth before mentioned, becomes a valuable curative agent. As occasional treatment, when the bowels are very inert, Dr. Garnett recommends injections of the water. He mentions that a course of the water very much tends to remove the troublesome symptoms of piles; and this seems probable, when we reflect how much that complaint depends upon obstruction in the circulation of the vena portarum; and upon costiveness. When the complaint, however, proceeds from, or is joined with, an irritated state of the mucous membrane of the rectum, the use of the water becomes more a matter of consideration.

Of cutaneous diseases, it is in the order squamæ of Willan, and the species lepra and psoriasis, that Harrogate water promises the most benefit. Dr. Willan gives his valuable testimony to its efficacy, when he remarks, " I have seen some very obstinate cases of lepra, alphos, and psoriasis, completely cured by the proper use of the waters of Harrogate."

I am led to believe that the water does not prove very successful in the different kinds of *acne;* and in the species rosacea, or gutta rosea of authors, it is apt to prove decidedly hurtful, seeming to aggravate the complaint by its heating influence on the stomach; for in this complaint the stomach is chiefly in fault, and very readily is inconveniently excited by stimulating fluid of any kind. I have met with cases of the acne punctata in which the most persevering trial has been given to the Harrogate water, almost without benefit. Dr. Bateman thus describes* this disease—" The eruption, in this variety of the disorder, consists of a number of black points surrounded by a very-slight raised border of cuticle. These are vulgarly considered as the extremities of small worms or grubs, because, when they are pressed out, a sort of worm-like appendage is found attached to them : but they are, in fact, only concreted mucus or sebaceous matter, moulded in the ducts of the sebaceous glands into this vermicular form, the extremity of which is blackened by contact with the air."

Harrogate water, as I have already stated, claims great regard as an alterative agent, independently of its purgative operation ; and this property appears to be due chiefly to its gaseous impregnation, which our analysis points out to consist not only of the sulphuretted and azotic gases, as stated by Dr. Garnett, but also of the carburetted hydrogen. In chronic obstruction of the liver, and of the spleen, a patient will visit Harrogate with almost certain advantage ; a mild mercurial oxide, with or without a purgative extract, according to the condition of the bowels, being used in conjunction with the water.

---

* Practical Synopsis of Cutaneous Diseases.

Dr. Armstrong, in his able work on scarlet fever, measles, consumption, &c. extols in very high terms the powers of Harrogate water, in many forms of chronic complaint. In the following account he speaks with great enthusiasm ; and, perhaps, may be said to generalise rather too much. " During a series of years, I have traced the operation of the sulphuretted hydrogen gas from one organ of the body to another ; from the skin, joints, and eyes, to the viscera of the head, chest, and belly : and the sum of my observation authorises me to declare, that it is one of the most powerful antiphlogistic agents which can be found ; for wherever the chronic inflammation be seated, it will more frequently remove it than any other single expedient which has hitherto been used and recommended by the medical faculty."

In other passages he alludes to the necessity of removing any active state of the inflammatory diathesis, as a preparatory step to the taking of the waters. On this point I have already offered my sentiments.

In gravel, the use of the water would in all probability be attended with much advantage. It acts very decidedly and very favourably as a diuretic. In cases of habitual deposition of lateritious sediment in the urine, I have witnessed the benefit which it has afforded.

## OF THE BATH.

IT appears to me that the same general principles which regulate the use of the ordinary warm bath, are applicable to the bath of Harrogate water, with, however, some additional caution. It is to be understood, as a preliminary to the employment of the bath, that the patient is properly prepared in those particulars relating to the constitution, which I have already stated, when speaking of the internal use of the water; for the action of this water is considerably stimulating to the surface, excites more than the common warm bath; and therefore it would be quite unsuitable in a feverish state of the habit. Dr. Garnett states in very positive terms, that the skin absorbs the water together with such substances as are dissolved in it; and asserts that, " besides the effects of the bath in cleansing the skin, and deterging the cutaneous vessels, a large quantity of medicated water is taken into the mass of blood, perhaps in a more active and less altered state than when taken in by the stomach." To discuss this question at length, would engage me in physiological arguments too extended for the present inquiry. I do not acquiesce in the latitude of the above opinion, but it is sufficient for our present purpose to know that the water used as a bath, has a very marked operation on the system ; more specific in its nature, than the simple warm bath. Enough, I conceive, is admitted to explain its effects, in considering that its strong impregnation with saline and gaseous matters, causes it to act very decidedly on the sentient surface of the body, and indirectly by sympathy upon the internal organs.

For those patients who are afflicted with cutaneous complaint, it will in most instances be advisable that the bath should be used at night, shortly before going to bed ; and that after being in bed, under circumstances when much freedom of perspiration is required, some warm diluting drink, as tea or gruel, should be taken. When a slight action only of the skin is wished, the patient may bathe at an earlier hour of the evening, and go to bed at his usual hour ; being careful, however, to avoid the night air.

In other disorders for which this bath may with much propriety be used, the proper time will be about an hour and a half before dinner, no unnecessary exercise being taken after bathing until the early part of the evening. The usual care of wiping the skin perfectly dry (so necessary in every kind of bathing), is to be duly observed ; and when the skin is the seat of complaint. very diligent friction should be used. The

degree of heat of the bath* will require some variation according to the temperament of the individual, and the nature of the complaint. The range will be from 93° to 97°, and 95° may be mentioned as the medium degree. When the bath is used for the cure of cutaneous complaint, the temperature should be 95° or 96°; and, for some patients 97° may be allowed. If used as a more general remedy to the constitution, or for the relief of gouty or rheumatic limbs, 95° will most commonly be the highest temperature that can be useful. The degree which is prescribed should be kept up during the whole time of the immersion; and the temperature should be determined by the thermometer, and not by the sensations of the individual. The stay in the bath will be ten minutes as the shortest, and twenty-five as the longest period; the longest time being allotted to the cases of cutaneous complaint; and the shorter to patients whose general state of constitution is delicate.

---

* We found by experiment that the best mode of retaining the gas in the water for the bath, is effected by mixing together one portion of the water boiling with another cold. This method succeeds much better than heating the whole of the water up to the temperature required for the bath. The water thus mixed gave almost as dark a precipitate with acetate of lead as the fresh water.

The frequency with which the bath is to be used, is another point of consideration. The repetition three times a week, or five times in a fortnight, may be stated as the average proper frequency. To use the bath two days in succession, and omit the third, will be the most frequent repetition, and twice a week the least, which, in this general kind of direction can be laid down as a rule.

The diseases requiring the employment of the bath, are all those which have been mentioned as proper for its internal administration; so that it is to be viewed as the auxiliary remedy. In addition to the complaints which I have already enumerated when speaking of the well, I may mention that a gouty and rheumatic state of limbs, strongly claims a trial of the bath. It is calculated to afford considerable relief in the sequelæ of these complaints, if used with judgment and discretion. It is inadmissible when decided gouty action is present or even threatened; and also when rheumatic inflammation, however slight, is affecting the limbs, in whatever texture such inflammation may be seated.

## OF MR. THACKERAY'S PUMPS.

The pumps belonging to Mr. Thackeray yielded a water so much of the same apparent strength as that of the Old Well, that it seemed desirable to examine their comparative degree of impregnation. We found that the water of the north pump, in particular, contained about the same proportion of sulphuretted hydrogen as the water of the Old Well, but the saline impregnation was considerably weaker. A third pump, very lately built, appears to furnish a water of equal strength with that of the north pump, as evidenced by the quantity of precipitate formed by the addition of a given quantity of sulphate of copper. Hence, therefore, although these pumps furnish a water more adapted to the purposes of bathing, than any of the other sulphuretted springs in Harrogate, they do not claim a right of equal regard with the water of the Old Well, as an internal remedy.

### OF THE CRESCENT WATER.

This spring, many years ago, was held in such estimation by Dr. Garnett, that he bestowed a separate Essay on its virtues. If the analysis of that chemist was correct, it follows, of necessity, that the spring has greatly degenerated in its properties. Dr. Garnett, represented its specific gravity as 1·002; that one gallon contained of sulphuretted hydrogen gas 13·6 cubic inches, and of carbonate of iron 2 grs. I derived the following results from my examination :

Its temperature was 52·5.

The specific gravity, 1·0008.

The smell of the water, its taste, and the effect of the acetate of lead applied as a test, concurred to shew that it was but weakly impregnated with sulphuretted hydrogen gas. Its low specific gravity is alone a proof of a slight impregnation with solid ingredients. Muriate of barytes produced a slight cloud. The tincture of galls indicated the presence of a small proportion of iron ; but, as a proof of the minute quantity, prussiate of potash scarcely produced an effect.

## OF ODDY'S SALINE CHALYBEATE.

This water is, unquestionably, the second in importance among the various springs of which Harrogate has to boast. It is obtained for drinking by means of a pump, the whole arrangement of which is very neat ; but, certainly, for the use of the invalid it is much to be desired that the water should rise from the spring into an open bason, having an aperture in its side for the excess of water to flow away. At present the water is very commonly pumped up in a flaky state, in consequence of the deposition of its iron in the bucket.

Its taste is strongly chalybeate, and also considerably, yet agreeably, saline.

Its temperature 54°.

The specific gravity of the water at 54°, was 1.0053, but at 60°, 1·0046.

### Action of Tests.

Litmus paper was slightly reddened, the blue being restored as it dried.

Turmeric paper, and that stained with the wild hyacinth, did not undergo any change of colour.

Acetate of lead produces a considerable precipitate, perfectly white in appearance.

Tincture of galls, an immediate lilac colour, which soon becomes intense.

Prussiate of potash, instantly a light blue, which in a few minutes deepens into azure blue. This and the preceding test produce no apparent change on the boiled water.

Solution of soap is slightly curdled.

Lime water is rendered milky.

Carbonate of ammonia produces a cloud, and by the addition of phosphate of soda a considerable precipitate forms, which is both granular and flaky.

Pure ammonia, and subcarbonate of soda, each a cloud.

Oxalate of ammonia, a dense cloud.

Nitrate of silver, an abundant precipitate.

From the action of these re-agents, we infer that the water contains magnesia, lime, and iron, combined with muriatic, sulphuric, and carbonic acids.

## ANALYSIS OF THE WATER.

My time at Harrogate did not permit the opportunity of making the necessary series of experiments, to determine with precision the properties of the gaseous ingredients of this water; but I may state, that the result of two experiments gave, for the wine gallon, of carbonic acid 10 cubic inches.

A.　One quart of this water was slowly evaporated to dryness in a glazed porcelain basin.

B.　The saline residue was digested in six times its weight of distilled water, in order to dissolve the salts soluble in that fluid, and this last solution was evaporated to dryness. The portion insoluble in water was put by for further examination.

C.　The saline compound obtained in the last process was digested with the assistance of a gentle heat in alcohol, of the specific gravity 815. The alcoholic solution was evaporated to dryness, and a deliquescent saline mass was obtained, which, by exposure to the atmosphere, became almost entirely dissolved.

D. The deliquescent mass was completely dissolved in distilled water, and the solution, when at a boiling heat, was decomposed by the addition of a sufficient quantity of subcarbonate of soda; the precipitate procured in this way, consisting of the carbonates of lime and magnesia, was thoroughly edulcorated by repeated portions of distilled water.

E. The precipitate obtained in the last process was treated with sulphuric acid, and a precipitate of sulphate of lime was formed, equivalent to $5\frac{1}{2}$ grs. of muriate of lime, and by decomposing the sulphate of magnesia, which was also formed in this process, by subcarbonate of soda, 2·2 grs. of carbonate of magnesia were produced, equivalent to 2·475 of muriate of magnesia.

F. The fluid remaining in process (e) was neutralized by nitric acid, and nitrate of silver was dropped in so long as any precipitate continued to be procured. The precipitate thus formed when dried at 212° weighed 32 grs. equivalent to 7·9 grs. of chlorine, leaving an excess of 2·57 grs. of chlorine beyond that proportion which is necessary to saturate the lime and magnesia obtained in the former process (d), and representing 4·3 grs. of muriate of soda.

G. The saline residue from which the alcoholic solution was separated in process (c) was dissolved in distilled water, and the solution divided into two equal portions. The one half was decomposed by the addition of nitrate of silver, and a quantity of muriate of silver was precipitated, which, when collected and dried, weighed 86 grs. equivalent to 35·4 of muriate of soda. Small quantities of the other portion of watery solution were assayed by nitrate of barytes, and by oxalate of ammonia. A slight cloud was produced by each of these re-agents. To the remaining portion, therefore, nitrate of barytes was added until it ceased to disturb its transparency. By this treatment ·4 of a gr. of sulphate of barytes was obtained, equivalent to ·2325 of sulphate of lime.

H. The insoluble residue left in process (b) was digested in dilute acetic acid, by which means a partial solution was effected, and this solution, when decomposed by subcarbonate of soda, yielded a white earthy precipitate. This, by subsequent treatment with a boiling solution of oxalate of ammonia, gave 2·4 grs. of oxalate of lime; and the remaining fluid was evaporated to dryness. The solid residue was heated to redness, dissolved in muriatic acid, and then precipitated by subcarbonate of soda, whence ·2 of a grain of carbonate of magnesia was obtained.

The residue insoluble in acetic acid was acted upon by muriatic acid, and the muriatic solution was decomposed by the addition of pure ammo-

nia, ·6 of a grain of oxide of iron was thus obtained.

A small portion of matter, amounting to ·1 of a gr.
insoluble in muriatic acid, was digested in a boiling solution of bi-carbonate of potash ; and when
this solution was decanted from it, nitric acid was
added ; but no solution could be effected in this
way. It was then boiled in a solution of caustic
potash, in a silver crucible, to dryness, and the
dry mass when treated by muriatic acid became
nearly all dissolved. By subsequent evaporation,
and washing with distilled water, a light gritty
precipitate separated, which had all the characters
of siliceous earth.

From those results, the composition of the
water in its solid contents may be stated as follows: In a wine gallon*

|  | Grains. |
|---|---|
| Of muriate of soda | 300·4 |
| —————— lime | 22 |
| —————— magnesia | 9·9 |
| Sulphate of lime | 1·86 |
| Carbonate of lime | 6·7 |
| —————— of magnesia | ·80 |
| Oxide of iron | 2·40 |
| Residue, consisting chiefly of silex.. | ·40 |
|  | 344·46 |

* Dr. Adam Hunter, of Leeds, published an Analysis of

Or, stating the composition according to Dr. Murray's views, the following results will appear:

| | Grains. |
|---|---|
| Muriate of soda | 291·5 |
| ———— lime | 29·35 |
| ———— magnesia | 10·80 |
| Sulphate of soda | 1·94 |
| Carbonate of soda | 8·07 |
| Oxide of iron | 2·40 |
| Residuum, consisting chiefly of silex | ·40 |
| | 344·46 |

this water last year, and the following is his tabular statement respecting the solid ingredients. In a wine gallon,

| | | |
|---|---|---|
| Muriate of soda | 434 | ·00 |
| ———— lime | 30 | ·00 |
| ———— magnesia | 13 | ·00 |
| Sulphate of lime | 9 | ·00 |
| Carbonate of iron | 5 | ·00 |
| ———— lime | 3 | ·00 |
| Loss | 2·50 | |
| | 496·50 | |

# MEDICAL HISTORY.

The analysis of this water will at once serve to shew, that its properties are alterative and tonic in a high degree. It appears to me to be a water possessing an excellent combination of saline ingredients, and of oxide of iron held in solution by carbonic acid.

The muriates of lime and magnesia are substances of decided medicinal power, and are contained in the water in sufficient proportion to be allowed the claim of efficacy; while the iron is even in rather larger proportion than in the chalybeate water of Tunbridge Wells. In most instances, however, when desiring the full action of a carbonated chalybeate, I should be disposed to give the preference to the spring of Tunbridge Wells, on account of its slight impregnation with other ingredients, and its greater consequent capability of acting as a chalybeate medicine.

I would offer the same general rules for the use of this water as for that of Tunbridge Wells, and therefore refer the reader to p. 75. I advise that the patient take this water as a chalybeate, and that he increase the doses according to the degree of tonic and exciting action produced on the

stomach and general system; not looking to its aperient effect upon the bowels: for, if he proceeded
with such a view, he would indiscreetly be taking too large a quantity of the iron. I repeat that
the principle on which the doses of the water are
to be increased, is, with entire reference to its
action as a chalybeate stimulant. It is true that
this water, from the presence of its muriates, will
not probably have the same restringent effect as
the more simple chalybeate of Tunbridge Wells,
yet it may require the aid of medicine for the
purpose of regulating the bowels; and this aid
will in general be most usefully lent by the employment of some suitable pill at bed time.

I have already stated that the Crescent water
appears to have undergone, in the course of years,
a remarkable change in its properties, being now
very weak both in its chalybeate and saline impregnation, and scarcely in any degree sulphuretted. If, therefore, it be desired to prescribe
the conjoined use of the sulphuretted and the
chalybeate waters, this plan will be happily ac-
complished by desiring the patient to visit the
Old Sulphur Well in the morning before breakfast, and this saline chalybeate spring in the
middle of the day, the relative quantities of the
waters being a point to be determined by the medical adviser, according to the nature of the case.

## ODDY'S PURE CHALYBEATE.

Close adjoining to the pump which yields the saline chalybeate, just now under consideration, a very pure spring has been discovered which is simply chalybeate. Last year, and I believe this to be the case at the present time, the water was not confined by any artificial arrangement, but presented itself freely rising up in a slight excavation made in the earth. The following concise description of its general properties appears to me sufficient.

Its temperature is 55°.

The specific gravity at 60°, 1·0003.

Its taste distinctly, yet not very strongly, chalybeate.

### Action of Tests.

Tincture of galls immediately produces a light purple, which in a few minutes deepens considerably. Prussiate of potash immediately occasions a light blue, which, in a few minutes becomes rather stronger in its tint, but not deep. No effect takes place from these tests in the boiled water.

Nitrate of silver produces a slight cloud.

Muriate of barytes, a slight cloud.

The moderate action of the two last re-agents, and the low specific gravity of the water, concur to shew that it is to be considered as a pure chalybeate; the iron being held in solution by carbonic acid.

I do not consider that the proportion of iron can exceed a grain and a half in the gallon; and I conceive this to be an extreme statement of the quantity*.

---

* I read with great surprise Dr. Hunter's statement, that this water contains ten grains and a half of carbonate of iron in the gallon, which is double the quantity possessed by the most active carbonated chalybeate, of which we have any knowledge. It appears to me that the above proportion is incompatible with the specific gravity of the water, which I examined twice, immediately at the spring. I regret the necessity of differing so widely from a fellow-labourer in the same vineyard. I made my investigation at the end of September, a period of the year when I have always found the water of Tunbridge Wells to be most strongly impregnated. I think it probable that some fallacy might have arisen with Dr. Hunter, from the circumstance of the water being always turbid, more or less, holding flakes of carbonate of iron in mechanical suspension; and unless the water is instantly passed through a filter, the mistaken result of an analysis is obvious. I would take the liberty of directing a similar observation to Dr. Hunter's analysis of the saline chalybeate, which he states to yield 5 grs. of the carbonate of iron for the gallon. This water is very commonly pumped up flaky, and requires the filter. Except in the errors which I must believe to belong to the analysis of these two waters, Dr. Hunter has written an able and entertaining essay.

### OF THE OLD SPA.

This spring is situated at Upper Harrogate, near the Granby Hotel, and is enclosed by a building which serves all the purpose of security from weather, and is sufficiently commodious. The water has a pleasant chalybeate taste, of moderate strength.

The temperature of the water is 54°.

Dr. Garnett states the specific gravity as 1·0014.

### *Action of Tests.*

Litmus paper receives a reddish tint just perceptible.

Paper stained with the wild hyacinth is not changed.

Tincture of galls instantly produces a violet hue, which soon becomes a light purple.

Prussiate of potash is immediately, yet very slightly, affected. The blue tint is not deep*.

---

* At the present time, August 9th, I have examined the chalybeate water of Tunbridge Wells, with galls and prussiate of potash. The colour from the former re-agent is an intense purple ; from the latter, a deep Prussian blue. The supply of the water is one gallon two pints and a half in a minute. The water, therefore, is not in its highest state of impregnation. See p. 68.

Solution of soap scarcely disturbs its transparency.

Nitrate of silver produces a slight cloud.

Muriate of barytes in a short time renders the water slightly turbid.

It is evident, from these experiments, that this water is very pure in its general composition, and that it has not a strong chalybeate impregnation. I should presume that it would be found to contain scarcely more than a grain of oxyd of iron in the gallon.

## OF THE TEWIT WELL.

This spring is situated in the forest of Knaresburgh, at a short distance from Upper Harrogate. It appears to have been discovered in the year 1571, and is recorded to have been the only mineral water known in the neighbourhood for a considerable time. It was named Tewhet or Tewit Spa, from the great number of lapwings which formerly frequented that part of the forest. The distance of the spring not being so convenient to the visitors of Harrogate as the Old Spa, it is now seldom used. Its properties are precisely similar to those of the Old Spa. Dr. Garnett allows it a very minute proportion more of oxide of iron in the gallon; but the difference is too inconsiderable to deserve notice; and I have merely given this brief sketch, that I might not make an omission in the list of Harrogate waters.

Although this distant part of the North occasionally presents the appearance of much wildness of country, yet Harrogate and its vicinity can boast of a great share of interesting scenery; and there are many objects of curiosity to tempt the visitor to make daily excursions. The air is bracing, and seems well suited to improve the health of the invalid; who may visit Harrogate with the fullest confidence in finding sulphuretted and chalybeate springs, of superior pretensions.

# BATH.

Bath is situated 107 miles west from London, and 12 east of Bristol. This ancient and elegant city is singularly favoured by Nature and Art, whose joint co-operations have conspired to give it importance and celebrity. The beauty and peculiarity of its situation are perhaps unequalled by any town in England. Planted originally in the bottom of a deep and narrow valley, it continued for ages to be confined to the dimensions which the Romans had first marked out; and, till within the last century, the ancient Roman walls (inclosing a space of about fifty acres) formed the boundaries of Bath. But the fashion and celebrity which it latterly obtained, induced many builders and speculators to extend the streets in all directions, by additional houses, which were instantly occupied upon completion.

The country round Bath consists of lias and *oolite* limestone. With this latter the houses in Bath are constructed. They are remarkable for their exterior neatness and beauty, and being raised over the sides of the broad acclivity of Lansdown (which rises to the north) in irregular groups of streets, squares, parades, circuses, and crescents, they present to the eye an appearance equally singular, magnificent, and beautiful*.

The climate of Bath, like that of the whole of this side of the kingdom, is in general very mild and genial ; an advantage which is however somewhat counterbalanced by the inconvenience of a larger proportion of rain than falls on the eastern part of our island.  The new town, indeed, from the great irregularity of its site, and the roughness of its soil, is very soon dry after the heaviest showers ; but then it is exposed to all the west and south-west winds, which here most prevail.  The lower part of the city is more sheltered by the adjacent hills.

The mineral springs of Bath are the only natural waters which we possess that are at all hot to the touch ; all the other thermal waters being of a heat below the animal temperature, and only deserving that appellation from being invariably warmer than the general average of the heat of common springs.  These waters, which have at first given celebrity to this spot on the banks of the Avon, and have been the means of erecting and supporting a splendid city, have long been eminently accommodated to the use of invalids

---

* Most of these observations are quoted from Rees's Encyclopædia.  See article Bath.

by the construction of elegant baths, pump rooms
for the drinking of the water, and various other
buildings calculated for convenience or amusement.

There appear to be three principal sources
of these waters, called the King's Bath, the Cross
Bath, and the Hot Bath. These springs all arise
within a short distance from each other, at the
lower part of the town, and not far from the
Avon, into which the hot water flows, after having
passed through the several baths. The supply of
water is so copious, that all the large reservoirs
used for bathing are filled every evening with
water fresh from their respective fountains.

The sensible properties of the Bath water are
the following. When first drawn it appears quite
clear and colourless, and remains perfectly quiet,
without sending forth any bubbles, or giving any
sign of briskness or effervescence. On standing
exposed for some hours it becomes somewhat turbid by the separation of a pale yellow ochrey
precipitate, which gradually subsides. The taste
of the water deserves particular attention, from
some peculiarities that attend it. When hot from
the pump, it fills the mouth with a strong chalybeate impression, without any particular pun-
gency, and accompanied with scarcely any kind
of saline taste. On this account it is by no means
disagreeable, and may be taken in a larger
draught without disgust than most other waters

K

in which the taste of iron predominates. As soon, however, as the water cools, even before any distinct precipitation appears, the chalybeate taste is entirely lost, and nothing but the slightest saline sensation to the tongue remains ; or rather, there is then no distinguishing difference between this and common hard spring water*.

The specific gravity of the three waters, the King's Bath, the Hot Bath, and Cross Bath, at 60°, examined by Mr. Children and myself in London, was found to be as follows :

Hot Bath.............1002·45
King's Bath† ...........1002·38
Cross Bath............1002·31

Mr. R. Phillips, whose elaborate analysis of the Bath water deserves particular regard, presents the following account of the temperature of the springs—" At the Hot Bath it is 117° ; at the King's Bath 114° ; and at the Cross Bath 109°.— This statement does not exactly agree with what has been usually given as their temperature. These results were obtained by pumping the water upon the bulb of a thermometer till the mercury ceased to rise." He observes, " that the springs may be considered as derived from one

---

* I have borrowed these introductory observations from Dr. Saunders's Treatise.

† Mr. Phillips gives the specific gravity of the King's Bath, 1002.

source, the temperature varying by their more or less circuitous passage to the surface."

I found, in my examination of the three waters, precisely the same kind of effect from re-agents, and differing only in degree ; the Hot Bath affording rather more evidence of impregnation than the King's Bath, and both these more than the Cross Bath ; a difference very well corresponding with the slight distinction of their specific gravity. I shall however follow Mr. Phillips's example, and confine my description to the effects produced on the water of the King's Bath.

No change is produced by the fresh water* either upon litmus paper, or that stained with the wild hyacinth.

Nitrate of silver produces a dense cloud.

Muriate of barytes, an immediate precipitate.

Oxalate of ammonia, an immediate dense precipitate.

Subcarbonate of soda, a dense cloud, quickly forming a flaky precipitate.

---

* With respect to the indications of iron in the water, I quote the following experiments from Mr. Phillips:

" Prussiate of potash, no immediate effect: after some weeks the water became slightly green.

" Tincture of galls, immediately a peach-blossom red colour, and very soon a precipitate, which became dark purple by exposure to the air."

Pure ammonia immediately renders the water milky.

Carbonate of ammonia produces a dense precipitate.—This was allowed to subside, and the liquor was filtered. Phosphate of soda was added to the clear fluid, and a granular precipitate, which partly adhered to the sides of the tube, slowly formed.

From the effects of these re-agents we are led to the conclusion, that the water contains sulphuric and muriatic acids, united to lime and magnesia ; and a small portion of oxide of iron held in solution by carbonic acid, as stated by Mr. Phillips. The unexpected circumstance of finding the evidence of magnesia in the water, which Mr. Phillips states as not existing in it, naturally surprised me very much, and I felt the immediate necessity of extreme care in calling in question the authority of a chemist so justly distinguished. In conjunction with Mr. Garden, I instituted the following examination. Half a pint of the water was evaporated to dryness. The residuum was submitted to the action of alcohol, in order that the muriates soluble in that menstruum might be dissolved. The alcoholic solution was evaporated. The solid matter was dissolved in distilled water, and then tested with pure ammonia, oxalate of ammonia, and the joint action of carbonate of ammonia and phosphate of soda. Oxalate of ammonia just produced a cloud ; but the other re-agents afforded the most irresistible evidence of an abundant proportion of magnesia.

Still determined to be sceptical of our results, for the reason already mentioned, I requested my friend Mr. Children to examine the water regarding the presence of magnesia. He adopted the following process; which I shall state in detail, as it was the method employed in the examination of all the remaining saline waters.

The water was first considerably reduced by evaporation, and the solid matter which became separated, was re-dissolved in very dilute muriatic acid, added in the least possible excess. The lime was then thrown down by oxalate of ammonia, and removed by the filter; very thin and pure paper being used. The clear liquor was evaporated to dryness, and the solid residuum exposed to a red heat, till the excess of oxalate of ammonia was entirely driven off, and the charcoal burnt away. The remaining salt was then re-dissolved in dilute muriatic acid, and the magnesia thrown down in the state of triple phosphate, by first adding phosphate of soda, and then pure ammonia in excess*. The precipi-

---

* This succeeds better than the bi-carbonate, the lime being previously removed; as the carbonic acid of this salt prevents a considerable portion of magnesia from falling down, unless the whole be boiled. This process also appears, from

tate collected in the filter was dried (with the counterpoise paper) at any temperature between 212° and 220°, and weighed. As much was then scraped off the filter as could be conveniently collected, and heated red. From the quantity of phosphate of magnesia thus obtained, that which the whole quantity of precipitate in the filter would have afforded (could it all have been collected) was estimated ; and from this, the weight of magnesia ; assuming the equivalent of phosphoric acid to be 35·33, and that of magnesia 24·66; which numbers a previous experiment had proved to be correct. The fact that magnesia is contained in the water, and in a considerable proportion, being thus demonstrated, the only possible ground of doubt will belong to the question, whether the water was procured from the genuine source ? In reply to this very proper inquiry, I shall here take occasion to record my declaration, that in supplying myself with the necessary quantities of the waters from all the watering places treated of in this volume, I exercised the utmost possible caution,—the most conscientious and scrupulous care, that in every instance I should be favoured with the genuine water. Such solici-

---

comparative experiments, to be still more favourable to the recovery of the whole of the magnesia than the one usually employed of boiling the water with either of the carbonated alkalies.

tude in the security of my proper object, has placed me under much obligation to various medical friends resident at the respective places; and as it would be inconvenient to enumerate so large a list, I trust that they will accept this general acknowledgment, as a sufficient expression of my grateful sense of their obliging attention.

As the Bath waters, and all the remaining saline waters of which I have to treat, contain the same bases and acids, however differently combined, and therefore have required similar processes to be used, I shall, with a view to relieve my reader as much as possible from the dull details of chemical statement, mention, once for all, the method which has been adopted to separate the component parts of the water under examination, by means of precipitants, according to the plan of analysis recommended by Dr. Murray.

In most instances two ounces of water was the quantity employed, and this was not concentrated by evaporation unless the water was of such slight impregnation as to require this preliminary step. For the separation of the sulphuric acid, nitrate of barytes was employed; for muriatic acid, nitrate of silver; for lime, oxalate of ammonia; and with respect to magnesia, the process has been already described.

The usual laborious care of washing the precipitates, drying them at 212°, and weighing them in a delicate balance, was of course observed. The composition of each water was estimated upon the following data:

Chloride of silver, according to Dr. Woolaston's scale, viz. 100 parts = to 24·62 chlorine.

Sulphate of barytes, according to ditto, viz. 100 parts = 34·01 sulphuric acid.

Oxalate of lime, according to a recent experiment of Dr. Marcet, viz. 100 parts of oxalate of lime, dried at 212° = to 39·23 of pure lime*.

The calculations for magnesia have already been fully stated.

It is quite obvious that an examination of so many waters by the direct mode of analysis, would have demanded the undivided time and attention of a practical chemist. The indirect mode by means of precipitants, serves every useful purpose for obtaining a medical knowledge of a water, if even it should not be thought the most eligible for perfect chemical accuracy. Certainly the mode of estimate so ingeniously pointed out by Dr. Murray, is admirably favourable to the consideration of a mineral water as a medical remedy. When, by means of the direct mode of analysis, a water yields sulphate of lime and muriate of soda, and not muriate of lime, the inference is drawn by Dr. Murray that these ingredients are in part the result of double decompo-

---

* See Phil. Trans. for 1819, part ii. p. 196.

sition, and that to some certain extent, more or less, the elements of the salts existed in the water, as sulphate of soda and muriate of lime. Hence the Physician is led to very different and important conclusions on the subject of the water as a medicine; the muriate of lime being a valuable medicinal agent; the sulphate of lime not entitled to any such praise; and the sulphate of soda, however minute in quantity, lending some useful aid. Dr. Murray has illustrated the whole view of the question very ably, and I shall content myself in this place with thus briefly adverting to his opinions, resuming here my more immediate subject.

The King's Bath water, therefore, analysed by precipitants, and stated upon the principle just now detailed, yielded the following results as to its saline contents* :—in a pint, or 16 ounces, as the mean of two experiments ;

Muriate of lime.............1·2
————— magnesia.........1·6
Sulphate of lime............9·5
————— soda ............ ·9

Mr. Phillips not only made an accurate esti-

---

* The quantity of residuum obtained from one pint of the King's Bath water, dried at 212°, was found, by two experiments, to be exactly 16 grs.; which quantity, according to Mr. Phillips, loses 2 grs. when dried at a red heat. Some of this loss must doubtless be referred to the escape of carbonic acid, but the greater part to the escape of water.

mate of iron in the water, but has also given an elaborate experimental dissertation on the influence produced by the presence of carbonate of lime upon the indications of iron effected by tincture of galls and prussiate of potash. He represents that the effect of tincture of galls upon the protoxide of iron is heightened by the joint action of carbonate of lime ; but, of prussiate of potash, that it is weakened.

The existence of silica in the Bath water was first detected by Dr. (now Sir G. S.) Gibbes; but the quantity which he describes it to contain was much larger than is assigned by Mr. Phillips ; the former gentleman making it nearly four grains in the quart, the latter only four-tenths of a grain.

Respecting the gaseous contents of this water, I shall take the liberty of quoting Mr. Phillips's results. The gas which rises in the form of bubbles through the water, and with considerable freedom, he found to consist of one hundred parts, of carbonic acid 5, azote 95 ; but by careful experiment he ascertained that the water did not contain any azote in solution ; a fact which we might readily expect when we consider the high temperature of the waters of Bath, and how loosely this gas is held by water in solution, unless at a lower temperature.

Borrowing, therefore, from a part of Mr. Phillips's analysis, the complete chemical view of the water will be as follows :—

In a pint,

Carbonic acid . . . . . . . . . . . . . . 1·2 *Cubic Inches.*

Grains.

Muriate of lime . . . . . . . . . . . . 1·2
——————- magnesia . . . . . . . . 1·6
Sulphate of lime . . . . . . . . . . 9·5
——————— soda . . . . . . . . . . ·9
Silica . . . . . . . . . . . . . . . . . . . . ·2
Oxide of iron . . . . . . . . . . . . . ·01985*
Loss, partly by carbonate of soda† ·58015

14

## MEDICAL HISTORY.

To embrace within the small limits which
the allotted space in this Treatise allows, the character of a water which has already filled whole

* About ⅛ of a gr. in a gallon.

† It will be obvious, that by the method which we adopted
by precipitants, we did not obtain the carbonates. Hence
part of the loss may be fairly referred to soda, or rather carbonate of soda, which would be obtained as carbonate of lime
by Mr. Phillips in the direct mode of analysis. The tabular
view given by this chemist is as follows:

| In a pint | Grains. |
|---|---|
| Sulphate of lime . . . . . . . . . . | 9·3 |
| Carbonate of soda, . . . . . . . . . | 3·4 |
| Sulphate ————- . . . . . . . . . | 1·4 |
| Carbonate of lime . . . . . . . . | ·8 |
| Silica . . . . . . . . . . . . . . . . . . . . | ·2 |
| Oxide of iron . . . . . . . . . . . . . | ·01985 |
| Error . . . . . . . . . . . . | ·11985 |

15

volumes, would be impossible; but I shall endeavour to give a clear outline of its properties and uses, and I am induced to do this the more particularly from having discovered the presence of magnesia in the water as one of its most considerable, and I may add one of its most important, ingredients.

The King's Bath water is the one most commonly employed in drinking. It is rather more strongly impregnated with magnesia than the Cross Bath, as the statement of our results will shew; but it appears to be not quite equal in this respect to the Hot Bath; and the three springs are evidently waters precisely of the same nature, but differing to the extent mentioned at p. 130, in temperature; and slightly in the degree of their impregnation. In the medical remarks which I have to offer, I wish to be understood as speaking of the King's Bath pump, to which the most usual resort is had. In the order of my subject, I have first to enter upon the internal use of the water.

I shall endeavour to discuss briefly the medical character of the water, in reference to its chemical composition, before I present any details founded upon its known operation.

In its gaseous impregnation, its power cannot be active; for it does not, as was stated by Dr. Saunders, contain azote in solution, and its proportion of carbonic acid is small.

In judging of the medicinal nature of the solid contents, as resulting from Mr. Phillips's ana-

lysis by the direct mode, we should be restrained
from ascribing any useful, certainly any considerable, influence to a single substance except the
iron ; but upon Dr. Murray's views, the water
will acquire higher pretensions. In his calcula-
tion he gave to a pint of the water 3·1 gr. of muriate of lime\*, and raised the proportion of sulphate of soda from 1·5 gr. to 5·5 gr. Dr. Murray's observations on the probable agency of the
muriate of lime, taken into the stomach with all
the advantages of minute division, and the aid of
temperature in the solvent, are so truly applicable to my present purpose, that I cannot forbear from making the following quotation :

" Muriate of lime, it is well known, is a substance of considerable power in its operation on
the living system ; in quantities which are even
not large, it proves fatal to animals. When taken
to the extent of six grains, the quantity of it
which, according to the preceding view, exists
in a quart of the Bath water, it cannot be inactive.
It is very probable, too, that a given quantity of
it will prove much more active in a state of great
dilution in water than in a less diluted form, as
in this diluted state it acts, when received into
the stomach, over a more extended surface ; and
besides this, whatever effect may be due to the

---

\* Dr. Murray did not know of the existence of magnesia
in the water. If the whole of the muriatic acid were supposed
to be combined with lime, the muriate of lime would be almost
accurately 3·1 grs. ; according to my present analysis.

high temperature of the Bath water in aiding the operation of the minute portion of iron it contains, the same effect must be equally obtained in aiding the operation of the much larger quantity of muriate of lime. The conclusion, indeed, as to the importance of this effect, is much more probable with regard to the muriate of lime than to the iron ; for supposing the quantity of the former to exist in the Bath water which has been assigned, the dose of it taken in a quart of the water is not far from its proper medium dose, and is at least equal to one-half of the largest dose which can be given, and continued without producing irritation ; while the dose of the iron is not the one-hundredth of that which is usually prescribed. Under the circumstances, therefore, in which the muriate of lime is presented in the Bath water, it is reasonable to infer that it must be productive of considerable immediate effect.

" The speculation is further not improbable, that, to produce its more permanent effects on the system as a tonic, it is necessary it should enter into the circulation. In a dilute state of solution it may pass more easily through the absorbents ; while in a more concentrated state it may be excluded, and its action confined to the bowels. Hence, the reason, perhaps, that in some of the diseases in which it is employed, scrofula particularly, it has frequently failed, its exhibition having been in doses too large, and in too concentrated a form. And hence it is conceivable that in a more dilute state, as that in which it may exist in the Bath water, besides its immediate operation, it may produce effects as a permanent tonic more important than we should otherwise expect.

Dr. Murray mentions, in confirmation of his opinion, that he " found a mineral water of considerable celebrity in Yorkshire, that of Ilkley, and which in particular was held in high estimation as a remedy in scrofulous affections by several eminent medical practitioners, to be water uncommonly free from all foreign matter, with the exception of very minute quantities of muriate of soda and muriate of lime." He had the opportunity of observing, at the same time, proofs of its medicinal efficacy.

In addition to this, the praise of the muriate of lime, I have now to introduce the muriate of magnesia, which, acting in conjunction with the muriate of lime *, may fairly be allowed some share of important action. Mr. Phillips describes the iron to exist in the water in the state of a protoxide; and this view I have no doubt is correct, and that in such state of oxidation it is held in solution by carbonic acid. This seems evident from the impossibility of detecting any indication of the metal after the boiling

---

* I can but consider that Dr. Murray may have over-rated the action of the muriate of lime. Otherwise, several of the other waters of which I treat, must possess, in this respect, a very high power.

of the water, or ordinary exposure to the air. I am at a loss, therefore, to explain the following observation of Dr. Murray: " I may add, that the iron in the Bath water is probably not in the state of oxide or carbonate, as has been supposed, but in that of muriate."

Regarding, therefore, the composition of the water, as stated in my table, p. 139, we may, with confidence, allow it a high claim as a medicine; and it is but just to add, that the indifferent estimation in which many medical practitioners have held the character of the water as an internal agent, has been wholly founded upon erroneous and deficient information of its chemical composition.

The quantity of iron is so small, that except we view its power as being assisted by the circumstances already mentioned, minute division, and temperature of the water, we might be thought too credulous in assigning to it much active property. Having thus considered theoretically the medicinal qualities of the water, I proceed to inquire into the results which experience, that grand arbiter of every question, has shewn to be justly due to its high reputation.

Dr. Falconer published the third edition of his Practical Dissertation on the Medicinal Effects of the Bath Waters in 1807, and lay claim to an acquaintance of more than twenty years with their nature and mode of action. He has considered their application in chlorosis;

visceral obstructions ; palsy, and as produced by
various causes ; gout ; rheumatism ; colic of Poic-
tiers (the painters); hypochondriasis, hysterical
complaints ; St. Vitus's dance ; and lepra."

Sir G. S. Gibbes, in a Treatise on the Bath
Waters, in 1803, has written on its properties very
much in the same order of diseases. I shall endeavour to offer an epitome of the opinions of these
authors, with such comments of my own, as my
more limited experience and my general reasoning, derived from chemical investigation, can enable me to make.

In a separate dissertation upon any remedy,
an author is naturally led into a partial praise of
its efficacy.   Dr. Falconer has the following
strong passage on this point in his well-con-
sidered Preface.

" Those who have written specific treatises
on the virtues of particular remedies, have contributed much to mislead the opinions of man-
kind concerning their efficacy.   Medicinal substances seem to be selected rather as subjects of
panegyric, than of impartial examination. Sometimes unworthy motives, and at others the caprice of prejudice, joined with a sanguine disposition of mind, have contributed to cherish this
empirical presumption, and to corrupt the fountains of information derived from matters of fact,
nearly as much as those that spring from the
most fanciful theory. When we peruse the cases

which have been the subjects of such trials, we are apt to think the character of the favourite remedy fully established, until melancholy experience replaces it in its true station, by teaching us, that it is possible, by florid description, amplification of success, and suppression of unfavourable events and circumstances, to mislead almost as effectually as by advancing a positive falsehood."

He recommends the water* in those disorders of deficient nervous energy, which go under the general term of chachectic, and commences with an account of chlorosis. He found it, for the most part, a very successful remedy in this complaint, care being taken to avoid its employment when any feverish excitement, and especially if any hectic symptoms, should be present.

Sir G. S. Gibbes lends his testimony to the particular efficacy of the waters in this complaint.

It is obviously a very appropriate remedy; and its favourable action will be materially assisted by the judicious use of the baths, at a higher or lower temperature, as the temperament of the particular patient and the circumstances of the case shall suggest.

Of the use of the water in visceral obstructions, Dr. Falconer speaks rather in general terms,

---

* It is more usual to speak in the plural number, but I shall deviate from this rule, as I consider that I am treating of one and the same water, only a little varied in its different springs.

specifying its particular employment in " that hardness about the region of the liver, and sometimes of the spleen, which often succeeds intermittent fevers, and was formerly attributed to the too early administration of the Peruvian bark, but is now proved to be the consequence of the disorder, and not of the medicine; and frequently owing to the neglect of giving the remedy at the beginning of the complaint."

Sir G. S. Gibbes advises the use of the water in that condition of the liver in which its functions are remarkably inert from obstruction, unattended with any inflammatory action, and when the stomach is affected with dyspeptic symptoms, dependant upon general want of tone in the digestive organs. A degree of jaundice attends this state of disorder, and the stimulus of the water has the praise, from these authors, of exciting healthy action in these important viscera, in a remarkable manner.

I am induced to think that the propriety of employing the Bath water in visceral obstructions, and dyspepsia, demands, in every instance, the most careful consideration. It is incumbent on us to view this remedy in the light of an active stimulant as well as alterative. These authors have very properly interdicted its application under any symptoms of an inflammatory nature; but *obstruction*, as a general term, is, in my apprehension, almost an expression of objection; and

I would say that for the most part, the Bath water
should not be employed in complaints of the ab-
dominal viscera, while any absolute obstruction
is actually existing.  As a tonic remedy, after the
sufficient employment of regular medicines, it is
entitled to our best confidence.  It is always to
be considered in diseases of obstruction, that if
we stimulate the organs of circulation prematurely, it is more probable that we shall excite
diseased than healthy action.  It must be our
object to restore proper function before we can,
with any fair prospect of advantage, excite the
unhealthy organ or organs to a greater degree of
action ;—if action alone be considered.

In no state of complaint is this principle of
reasoning more applicable than in the treatment
of *palsy*.   Dr. Falconer and Sir G. S. Gibbes have
offered very clear and judicious instructions upon
the circumstances in this disease which authorise,
and those which forbid, the employment of the
water ; but no written general instructions can
supersede the strict necessity of a distinct investigation into the causes of symptoms in every individual case.  Do they proceed from apoplexy having actually preceded the paralysis, or from a condition of vessels bordering upon apoplexy ?—Do
they proceed from disease of structure in any part
of the vertebral column, or from disease in the spi-
nal marrow itself ? Or does an extreme atony exist
from the influence of causes which have impaired

the energy of the brain and nerves, and produced
a palsied state of some particular part of the body,
which may have been weaker than other parts in
its original conformation, and therefore more pre-
disposed to loss of healthy power?—From these
premises the obvious conclusion follows, that the
use of the Bath water is to be considered in the
character of an active stimulus, and is contra-in-
dicated except as a remedy for the remote effects
of the diseases just mentioned, and even then is to
be employed with every circumspection in regard
to the existence of remaining obstruction and plethora.   In dyspepsia, arising out of a studious
sedentary life, and from many other causes of
debility which might be mentioned (all circumstances of contra-indication being at the same time
considered), the stimulus of the water seems particularly applicable.

In those consequences of *gout* which are
marked by various signs of debility, the waters of
Bath have gained the reputation of being almost
specifically useful.   Dr. Saunders remarks, " In
gout the greatest benefit is derived from this
water in those cases where it produces anomalous
affections of the head, stomach, and bowels ; and
it is here a principal advantage to be able to
bring by warmth that active local inflammation
in any limb which relieves all the other troublesome and dangerous symptoms.   Hence it is that
Bath water is commonly said to produce the gout,

by which is only meant, that where persons have a gouty affection shifting from place to place, and thereby much disordering the system, the internal and external use of the Bath water will soon bring on a general increase of action, indicated by a flushing in the face, fulness in the circulating vessels, and relief of the dyspeptic symptoms ; and the whole disorder will terminate in a regular fit of the gout in the extremities, which is the crisis always to be wished for."

Dr. Falconer observes, " The Bath waters are well suited to that kind of gout called by Sauvages the winter gout, which is indeed the most common of any. This usually comes on towards the decline of life, and does not in general keep regular periods, but is subject to recur throughout the whole year, the summer months excepted." He adds, " this kind of gout is always attended with signs of weakness of the stomach and organs of digestion, such as imperfect concretions, and nervous irritations, flatulence and want of appetite."

Sir G. S. Gibbes has considered the use of the water both in gout and gravel.

In my Treatise on Gout I have entered upon further considerations on the use of the Bath waters in this disease than my present limits will allow, and I shall confine myself to a few observations.

I speak from sufficient experience in saying

that the Bath water, either employed internally or externally, is inadmissible, when an active state of gouty diathesis is present; when the tendency to relapse is strongly established in the constitution, whether from the use of Eau Medicinale, Wilson's Tincture, Reynolds's Specific, or similar baneful medicines; or from continued irregularities in living. Also, when plethora; a state of circulation easily excited to inflammatory action; or marked obstruction in the vessels of the liver, are found to exist. As a general opinion I would venture to observe that a gouty patient should be restricted to any free use of the water, and perhaps to its employment altogether, unless debility of the stomach, or nervous system, unattended by gout, prevail; or unless that kind of chronic gout is happening in which it is to be desired that a fit, as it is called, should be excited for the relief of the constitution, which, under such circumstances, is oppressed with all the distressing symptoms of hypochondriasis. I must add, however, that cases of this description must be attentively studied, as to the question of visceral obstruction.

I would here beg to suggest, that when the Bath water is found to be too exciting in its effects, it should be tried as a stimulant alterative only, free from the more powerful influence which belongs to its chalybeate impregnation. Into such a remedy it is easily converted by taking the water after it has been exposed to the air for a few hours, and then warmed to any temperature which may be directed. In this state it will only have lost the oxide of iron and some of the carbonate of lime, and will retain the muriates, on which so much of its virtues may be stated to depend, in full proportion.

Mr. Phillips found that the water had lost all traces of iron in its composition after being allowed to cool.

In *rheumatism*, the Bath waters are admissible only in the chronic form of the complaint. The internal use of the waters will be no otherwise a remedy than as improving the tone of the stomach and general system, and thereby aiding its external employment, which I shall have to consider more particularly when speaking of the baths.

For the relief of the distressing consequences of the lead colic, commonly called the painter's colic, the Bath water, used both internally and externally, promises to be a valuable remedy. The restoration of tone in the muscular action of the bowels may probably be much assisted by its further daily employment as an injection. At the King's and Hot Baths, there is an apparatus for distending the intestines with the water by means of the pressure of a column of water; the fluid being propelled through a tube introduced into the bowels.

Hypochondriasis and hysteria being disordered states of the constitution of a secondary nature, and dependant on many different causes, the use of the Bath water for their relief cannot form the subject of my present consideration.

Dr. Falconer speaks rather favourably of its operation in several cases of St. Vitus's dance. He states " that bathing, and pumping the spine of the back moderately, twice or three times a week, seemed to be the principal circumstances that led towards a cure."

In lepra, the Bath water appears, from Dr. Falconer's report, to have been remarkably successful. The bathing in this disease is of the most importance; but the water internally may be expected to prove an active auxiliary.

Having given this rapid sketch of the principal disorders in which the Bath water appears to claim most regard, I shall conclude, before proceeding to the notice of the baths, with a few remarks on the method of drinking the water ; and shall avail myself of the experienced opinions of the authors already quoted.

Dr. Falconer states, that the waters when drunk fresh from the spring, " have in most persons the effect of raising and rather accelerating the pulse, increasing the heat, and exciting the secretions ; that they promote the action of the skin and of the kidnies, and are also found to increase the salivary discharges. Hence, he adds, they are found in cases where there is no tendency to fever, to quench the thirst better than any other fluid." He remarks, that " he has seen persons to whose stomachs they were particularly grateful and strengthening, who were debarred from their use even in small quantities, by their constantly exciting a fever after the use of them was commenced, although no apparent tendency to fever in the habit of the body had previously subsisted."

For such patients I strongly advise a trial of the water on the plan and principle which I have suggested at page 151.

Although so little material difference appears from chemical examination to exist in the three waters, yet it seems reasonable to take into consideration the influence of temperature, notwithstanding that, in the opinion of some, the difference of a few degrees more or less appears unimportant. It is a point which must be determined by experience.    In regard to the magnesian impregnation, the Hot Bath claims the preference.  The waters from the three pumps yielded by analysis, magnesia, which I describe as muriate of magnesia, in these comparative proportions; from a pint, Hot Bath, 2·5 grs. ; King's Bath, 1·6 gr. ; Cross Bath, 1·3 gr.

Each of the waters being tested with the tincture of galls and prussiate of potash, in August, produced just the same effects as described, p. 131 ; but the Cross Bath appeared to afford, in a very slight degree, the most evidence of

iron. Sir G. S. Gibbes remarks, that " the Cross
Bath water is generally considered to be the least
stimulating and heating of the three ; and that
the water of the Hot Bath pump appears less
stimulating than that of the King's Bath." He
adds, " I have known several patients, who have
been obliged to return to the use of the Cross
Bath water, after trying the water of the King's
Bath, in consequence of the feverish heat excited
by the latter ; and this, even though the smallest
glass of the King's Bath water had been substi-
tuted for the largest at the Cross Bath." Upon
this statement it would appear, that the influence
of higher temperature must be considered as the
cause of the difference in question. I should
certainly expect rather the highest exciting power
to be found in the water of the Hot Bath.

It must be laid down as a rule, that every
patient should consult his medical adviser as to
his fitness of preparation for entering upon a
course of the water. In saying this I am strictly
considering the welfare of the invalid, who cannot
possibly have any judgment whether the case
call for or allow the use of the water, or whether
it should be preceded by a little reduction of the
circulation by means of local or general bleed-
ing ; or what aperient medicines may previously
be necessary.

Sir G. S. Gibbes rather objects to Dr. Falconer's opinion, that the increase of the urinary
discharge is a good criterion that the waters agree.

He thinks that this indication is not to be relied upon, and that a stronger proof is derived from their occasioning a flow of saliva and allaying thirst.

Although I am convinced that no patient should enter upon the use of the Bath water without previously obtaining medical advice, I may briefly mention the usual doses in which it may be taken. Half a pint twice a day, drunk at two intervals; the first quarter of a pint an hour, or rather less, before breakfast, and the second at one or two in the day, may be described as the smallest quantity; and a pint and a half in divided portions, as the largest amount. In the use of this latter total quantity, the patient should subdivide the doses, using intermediate exercise for twenty or thirty minutes.

The regulation of the bowels by suitable means, the plan of regimen and diet, and the conjoining any medicine of a general nature with the use of the water, are further points of consideration which will engage the judgment of the medical adviser in every particular case, and do not require any general observations. I hasten therefore to some account

## OF THE BATHS.

THE public baths are three in number, the Hot, the King's, and the Cross Bath.

The temperature of the baths varies in different parts according to their proximity to the spring :—Thus the Hot, or Hetling Court Bath, near the spring, is about 106° ; the uniform heat of the general bath may be stated as 104°. The King's Bath, nearly over the spring, or within the circular railing, which is about two yards in circumference, 100°, and at the entrance 98°, which I believe to be the general standard heat of this bath. The Queen's Bath is in fact a part of the King's, separated by an arch, as two drawing-rooms are by folding doors, and its temperature is two or three degrees lower. The Cross Bath varies from 98° to 96°.

In dimensions, the Hot Bath is an octagon of about 21 feet in diameter. The King's is about 65 feet in length, and 40 in breadth. The Queen's is a square of about 25 feet in diameter. The Cross Bath is of irregular form, and somewhat larger than the Hot Bath. They are all about 4 feet 7 inches in depth.

Each bath has a contiguous pump-room. There are *douches* in the three public baths, and a separate douche, out of the bath, at the King's Bath. At the Hot Bath there are vapour and shower baths. The hospital patients and poor are generally sent to the Hot Bath ; but sometimes, when they require a bath of lower temperature, to the Cross Bath. The public baths are emptied daily ; the water which rises one day being discharged before the next, by drains into the river Avon. The Hot Bath re-fills in eight or nine hours; the King's and Queen's, in eleven hours; and the Cross in seventeen. Hence a support seems to be afforded to Mr. Phillips's opinion " that the springs may be considered as derived from one source, the temperature varying by their more or less circuitous passage to the surface." The King's Bath is stated to contain, when at its usual height, 346 tons, 2 hogsheads, and 36 gallons of water. The public baths, and a set of private baths, are the property, and under the direction of the corporation.

These private baths are eight in number: four at the King's, and four at the Hot Bath; they are each nine feet in length from the top of the steps to the other extremity of the bath; six feet six inches wide at the broadest part, and four feet seven inches in depth. Each contains about thirteen hogsheads of water. Those at the Hot Bath are rather the largest, and contain two or three hogsheads more than the King's private baths.

There is also another establishment of private baths, with a pump room, called the Kingston baths. These belong to, and are managed by an individual.

The temperature of the water at each bath from the dry pump, as it is called, is higher than that of the general bath. For example, at the Hot Bath it rises to 116°.

The water deposits in its progress to the baths, upon the pipes and other channels, a ferruginous precipitate. The springs also throw

out a pyritical looking sand.  Of this I made an
examination, and found it to be silex interspersed
with portions of carbonates of lime and iron, as
shewn by a considerable effervescence being produced on the addition of muriatic acid ; and the
solution yielding precipitates of iron and of lime,
by the action of ammonia, and oxalate of ammonia.  When ignited upon a piece of platina foil,
it here and there furnishes points of a pale blue
flame, yielding at the same time a distinct sulphureous smell.  This description of the properties of the sand may suggest some speculation as
to the heat of the water being caused by a chemical decomposition of sulphuret of iron in the
bowels of the earth ; for we know that caloric is
liberated in considerable abundance, in many instances where bodies undergo a change in their
state of combination.  But I must forbear from
engaging in so difficult a question.

A conferva, classed by Mr. Sowerby among
the minute warm spring confervæ, forms upon
the sides and bottom of the public baths, and
floats upon the surface of the water.  This author
in the 36th vol. of his English Botany, plate
2584, describes this conferva " as spreading rather unequally in broad velvet-like patches of a
dark green colour.  The irregularity of its appearance arises from the filaments being collected together with little ascending tufts apparently rooted in the muddy deposit of the water.

Each tuft proves, on examination, to consist of simple uniform even filaments crowded together, quite pellucid, and equally destitute of joints and branches. Their diameter is not more than 8 or 10,000 parts of an inch ; this being one of the most minute species that we have examined." I trust that these preliminary particulars of the baths will be found not uninteresting. I proceed to consider their *medical use.*

Dr. Falconer commences his account of the external use of the bath waters, by stating his opinion that they do not cause the relaxation produced by an ordinary warm bath. He remarks, " the Bath guides likewise, many of whom every morning remain several hours in the water, do not seem at all relaxed or weakened by such a practice, but on the contrary are in general robust, vigorous, and long lived, and most of them inclining to corpulency.

" Fainting, likewise, which a warm bath of common water is so apt to induce, happens very rarely in these baths, although the stay is generally longer than in a common warm bath, and the people who use it are often in a very weak state both of strength and spirits."

The opinion here expressed seems to me very reasonable, and more especially when we consider that the patient has the advantage of free space that he may keep up muscular action during the immersion.

The apartments are prevented from becoming oppressive, by the judicious use of ventilation. Dr. Falconer relates examples of the success of the baths in every kind of palsy, except when depending upon an apoplectic condition of the vessels of the brain. When speaking of palsy from lead, he quotes Dr. Charlton's account, that in two cases, " in one of which the bath was not tried until one-and-twenty months after the seizure ; and another, wherein seven months were elapsed after a second attack before the patient came to the bath ; yet, notwithstanding, both of them perfectly recovered."

Dr. Falconer has, in the course of his dissertation, extolled the power of the Bath waters, as a remedy in many disorders calling only for the occasional use of the ordinary warm bath. Not entering so fully into his panegyric, I shall pass over this extended view of the subject, admitting as a general argument, that when it suits the convenience of the individual, he would, under most circumstances when requiring the use of a warm bath, derive more comfort, and probably more advantage, from the free range of the warm bath at Bath, in preference to immersion in the ordinary confined warm bath. I shall limit my present view to the consideration of gout, rheumatism, and diseases of the bursæ mucosæ, as medicable by the use of the baths.

M

A gouty patient is not always precluded from making trial of the baths, even although the use of the water internally would be decidedly improper. Yet it holds, I think, as a general rule, that the water should not be employed in either mode when the system is in so susceptible a condition, that almost any exciting power serves to bring gouty irritation into action. From this statement must be excepted the instances in which the constitution is in a state of such general disorder, that some active and concentrated gouty action is desired ;—or, in other words, when a fit of gout is wanted. I have known many instances, in which the gouty disposition has been so strong, that one or two bathings have served to produce a paroxysm, even without the internal use of the water; but I must add, that such a consequence is not peculiar to the Bath water. A similar effect in such constitutions, or states of constitution, happens also from the common warm bath.

Dr. Saunders, indeed, has called in question the specific influence of the Bath water externally applied. He remarks, when speaking of the waters and of the convenience of the baths, " But its eulogists, not content with this, have affirmed, that even when used externally, it exercises a stimulant power on the skin, which renders it preferable to common water ;" and he proceeds with arguments attempting to shew that the only grounds of superiority are, agreeable temperature and the opportunity of keeping in free motion. I confess that I do not enter wholly into this scepticism. It appears to me very probable, that a water impregnated, as the water of Bath is found to be, should exercise some specific action on the sentient surface of the body, beyond that of common water raised to the same temperature. I shall beg therefore to assume this opinion as not incorrect, and proceed now with my medical discussion.

It will happen in some instances that it is expedient to use the waters internally without bathing, and in others to bathe only. Of the latter fact, I quote the following statement from an intelligent patient, as an illustration.

A gentleman, aged 55, robust and plethoric, first attacked with gout at the age of 29 (the disposition not hereditary), suffered a severe paroxysm in the beginning of autumn, which was regularly and successfully treated. In September, being quite convalescent, he went to Bath, as it was his occasional plan to do. He favoured me with the following statement: " After the usual preparation by aperient medicine, I commenced the drinking of the water of the Cross Bath, with one glass of the middling size before breakfast, and the same quantity before dinner. It agreed with me as usual on former occasions, always giving an excellent appetite, and an extraordinary flow of spirits. At the end, however, of eight

days, I began to feel the approach of gout very
sensibly in the feet, and in short was quite lame.
My physician considered that the water was too
stimulating, and advised its discontinuance. I
should remark, that I was not sensible of any
fever, and did not notice the usual discolouring
of my tongue, nor the appearance of the pink
sediment in my urine during this attack. After,
however, the swellings of the ankles had subsided, I was still distressed with flying pains
about them and my feet. I was next recommended to try the effect of the King's Bath, and
not to think of the internal use of the water. I
bathed in consequence every other day, and finding the plan agree, and that the pains in my feet
sensibly diminished, I continued it regularly five
weeks; and the result was very satisfactory indeed."

Both as regards the internal and external use
of the water, I am led to expect most advantage
from it to the gouty patient in cases of the chronic
form of the disease, in which there is great deficiency of nervous energy in the muscles, joined
with languid circulation in the extremities, and
stiffness with aching pains in the joints upon
every motion. In the example I am supposing,
the tendons are rigid and thickened, the ligaments are wanting in elasticity, and the bursæ
are distended. There is no external redness, the
feet are frequently cold, and in short the limbs

seem to want animation, and to require a high degree of stimulus.

If care be required by the gouty invalid in the use of the bath, still greater will be demanded in having recourse to the dry pumping, technically so called, from the circumstance of the rest of the body, except the part pumped upon, being kept dry.  It is more or less stimulating in its action, according to the degree of heat of the water and the force with which it is projected.  When the parts which have been weakened by gout are simply in a state of weakness and stiffness, the effect of pumping promises to be highly useful.  It is most certain to be successful under the advantages of freedom from all tendency to inflammatory action, or feverish state of the system.  Any marks of active gouty diathesis must be watched with every care ; for if there be much susceptibility to gouty action, the stimulus of pumping will be too great an excitement.

In chronic rheumatism the baths possess a high and well-merited reputation.  It must not be considered as a remedy of universal application in this complaint ; so various are its forms ; so much is it modified by individual tempera- ment and constitution.  Doubtless it will be found most useful in those cases in which the inflammatory diathesis is absent, and in which there is but little tendency to febrile irritation.  In this form of the complaint, for the most part, the patient, when sitting at rest, is free from pain, and suffers his distressing uneasiness only upon moving. The joints are stiff, and produce a harsh grating noise on being moved. This *grating* may probably be attributed to the comparatively dry and unhealthy state of the cartilaginous surfaces, and defective secretion of the synovial membranes. The bursæ mucosæ are distended and occasionally tender ; the tendons rigid and thickened. From the disorganized condition of the ligaments, and probably from absorption of the smooth surfaces of cartilages being attended with adhesive inflammation, or from earthy depositions in the joints, partial or complete anchylosis now and then takes place. It is obvious that any serious change of structure in this way is without remedy ; but it is equally clear that it may often be prevented by timely attention ; and many morbid conditions of the soft parts will certainly admit of materially useful treatment.

Dr. Falconer, speaking of chronic rheumatism, states as follows ; " In the space of five years (to wit), from the beginning of the year 1775, to the end of the year 1779), three hundred and sixty-two patients were admitted for this disorder into the Bath Hospital, of whom one hundred and twenty-seven were cured, one hundred and forty-four were much better, forty-two were better, forty-one were no better, and eight died, four of whom died of the small pox.

" The proportion of the number benefited, to

the whole number received into the hospital for this complaint, is as 313 to 362, or nearly as 1 to 1·156. The proportion of those benefited to those that received some benefit, is as 6·3877 to 1."

The bursæ mucosæ are liable to a distinct form of complaint from either gout or rheumatism, acquiring from a process of diseased secreting action, a state of enlargement, and either of remarkable softness or hardness, varying chiefly according to the size of the bursa which is affected. I am now adverting only to the chronic variety of this disease. There is seldom pain, but rather a sense of uneasiness and stiffness upon motion. The knee joint is most commonly affected, and produces most lameness ; but other joints, both in the upper and lower limbs become affected. The application of pumping is in this complaint almost specifically useful ; and I am not aware that much advantage is to be expected from the bathing as regards the bursæ only, but on other grounds, the general bath also will most commonly be proper.

Of the pumping, Dr. Falconer observes, " From fifty * to two hundred strokes is the number generally directed to be taken at one time, which may however be increased or diminished according to the age, sex, strength, or other circumstances of the patient. The pump likewise, as its application is partial only, may be properly

* In many cases I conceive it will be better to commence with thirty strokes only.

used of a greater degree of heat than a bath for
the whole body.

In regard to the season of the year, it seems
agreed on all hands, that hot and cold weather
are both objectionable, and spring and autumn
therefore are the most eligible periods.

For the time of using the bath, the following
observations of Dr. Falconer appear to me perfectly appropriate : " If the patient use the public
baths, it is necessary that he should go to them
before nine in the morning, as they are emptied
soon after that time ; but a much earlier hour is
generally chosen. If the private baths are preferred, they may be prepared at any time of the
day, and I am not certain that any particular hour
possesses advantages peculiar to itself. I have
known equal benefit gained in the morning, at
noon, and in the evening. Those who prefer
the latter hour, should be careful to dine rather
early, and to pay especial regard to moderation,
with respect to the quantity and quality both of
food and liquor."

Whether a bath of the highest temperature,
as the Hot Bath ; or of the lowest, as the Cross
Bath, shall be chosen, must depend wholly on
the case and on the individual constitution ; as,
also, the duration of the immersion.

In conclusion, I ought to state my opinion,
that when a temperature lower than 94 does service, the patient should be considered in a state
of preparation for Buxton. In having dwelt

upon the use of the Bath water as a remedy in the three complaints just considered, I have not intended to lose sight of the superior pretensions of the Buxton Bath for most conditions of these complaints.    Bath, I apprehend, deserves the preference only in that state of the limbs, in which the circulation is very languid, as shewn by coldness of the extremities; and remarkable stiffness constantly prevails, as described at page 166.

In all these complaints of the limbs, whether Bath or Buxton be the appointed place of resort, the patient should not fail to add to the baths, the important remedy of friction and champooing.   I must pass over, without further comment, the other disorders in which the use of the baths is said to be efficacious.   The authors above quoted have given a considerable list; and for more general information on the subject, I beg to refer the reader to their volumes.

# CHELTENHAM.

————

THE town is situated 94½ miles, by the Uxbridge road, W. N. W. from London. The various handsome buildings and elegant villas, which are continually rising up to adorn the place and neighbourhood, have already exalted Cheltenham and its charming environs to a high degree of beauty and importance.

Dr. Jameson * remarks, " The Valley of Evesham, now more frequently called the Valley of

———

* A Treatise on the Cheltenham Waters, and Bilious Diseases. The same author quotes from Cary the following account of the relative situation of Cheltenham to other places, considering it as the centre :

| | | |
|---|---|---|
| Gloucester.. ... | 9½ miles | S.W. |
| Bristol............ | 44½ —— | S.W. |
| Bath............. | 44½ —— | S.S.W. |
| Monmouth...... | 35 —— | W.S.W. |
| Worcester...... | 25 —— | N.N.W. |
| Malvern......... | 22 —— | N.W. |
| Tewkesbury... | 9 —— | N.W. |
| Oxford.......... | 40 —— | E.S.E. |
| Cirencester. ... | 16 —— | S.S.E. |
| Evesham........ | 16 —— | N.N.E. |
| Winchcomb... | 7 —— | N.E. |

Gloucester, is not excelled in beauty and sylvan
scenery, by any spot whatever, and derives vi-
vacity from the Severn winding in its centre, and
embellishment from the numerous rural villages
and plentiful orchards, which every where adorn
its surface."

As a geological description, I may state, that
the country immediately around Cheltenham consists of a blue clay, which is denominated Lias,
and which frequently contains beds of argillaceous
limestone. The Coteswold Hills, in its neighbourhood, are composed of calcareous rocks of
the bolitic kind.

## OF THE WATERS.

Whatever deficiency of springs may formerly
have existed at Cheltenham, no such fault certainly now prevails ; but, on the contrary, such is
the real or nominal variety, that it becomes a
task of no slight difficulty to give all the details
necessary to a clear and full information respecting the different wells.

I have to speak of the original spa, Thompson's
or Montpelier Spa, and the Sherborne Spa
Each is furnished with pump rooms of noble size
and elegance, with adjoining pleasure grounds.
Indeed, such are the excellent arrangements,
that the invalid, gladdened also by enlivening

bands of music which attend the morning promenade, is invited to fulfil his early duty of health by all the attractions of a gay and lively scene.

I have also to describe the two chalybeate springs.

### THE ORIGINAL SPA, OR OLD WELL.

It is so named from being the oldest mineral well at Cheltenham, accidentally discovered about a century ago. It is situated in the centre of a beautiful avenue of elm trees, not five hundred yards from the middle of the town. The analysis reported by Dr. Saunders in his General Treatise, 1800, refers only to one water (the present No. 1.); but now the numbers or kinds at this pump room are nominally four. I have been careful to ascertain the nature of the difference between these numbered waters.

Their temperature varies according to the season of the year. Thus the No. 3, in the latter end of the month of October 1819, was 43°, and at the end of May 1820, 53°. This account of the temperature applies to all the saline waters at Cheltenham.

### No. 1.

This is described on the proprietor's card, as the *strong ærated chalybeate saline,* and as the original spa. Its taste is mildly and pleasantly

saline, and not chalybeate. Its specific gravity*
is 1·0091.

## ACTION OF TESTS.

Litmus paper is just perceptibly reddened,
but that stained with the wild hyacinth does not
undergo any change †.

Lime water renders the water slightly milky.

Solution of soap produces a slight flaky precipitate.

Pure ammonia does not immediately impair
its transparency.

Muriate of lime, no change.

Subcarbonate of soda renders it slightly milky.

Carbonate of ammonia produces a slight cloud,
which is increased by the addition of phosphate
of soda.

Nitrate of lead, a considerable white precipitate.

Pure barytes, a dense cloud.

Muriate of barytes, an abundant precipitate.

Nitrate of silver, a copious precipitate.

---

* It is to be observed that the specific gravity of all the
waters at Cheltenham, was not taken at the spring, but
shortly after.

† For the sake of brevity, I may here note, that all the
other waters at Cheltenham acted on these papers without any
marked difference of effect.

Oxalate of ammonia, a dense cloud.

Tincture of galls, in a very feeble degree, indicates the presence of iron.

Prussiate of potash produces a very slight green tinge.

From these effects we may presume that the water contains lime and magnesia, and sulphuric and muriatic acids, a very minute portion only of iron, and an inconsiderable impregnation with carbonic acid.

### ANALYSIS BY PRECIPITANTS.

One pint, upon an analysis conducted on the principles already detailed, and calculated on the data* described at p. 136, afforded these results.

---

* I must not omit to notice, that the calculations for the Harrogate sulphuretted water. at p. 99, in regard to the muriates, was made upon the theory that they are real muriates, not chlorides, the equivalent for muriatic acid in such cases being chlorine + hydrogen. The calculations for all the other waters in this volume are formed upon Sir Humphrey Davy's original theory, that they are not muriates but chlorides ; consisting of chlorine and the metallic base ; as, for example, common salt consists of chlorine and sodium without water. Upon this supposition, the following will be the computation of the muriates in the Harrogate water, instead of that stated at p. 99 : muriate of soda, 734·82 grs. ; muriate of lime, 51·73 grs.; muriate of magnesia, 31·62. The number giving these results is upon Dr. Woolaston's scale, as mentioned at p. 136.

In a pint,                                            Grains.

    Muriate of soda.......58·20
    Muriate of lime........ 6·21
    ————— magnesia.... 2·54
    Sulphate of soda......14·56

              81·51

Oxide of iron, a minute portion.

### No. 2.

Described by the proprietor as the *strong sulphureous saline.*

Taste, saline and very slightly chalybeate ; the smell just perceptibly sulphuretted.

The specific gravity, 1·0089.

The effects of re-agents is precisely the same as described of No. 1, and, as with that water, tincture of galls slightly indicates the presence of iron ; the prussiate of potash produces a distinct shade of green. The title of the water would naturally lead us to expect a considerable impregnation with sulphuretted hydrogen ; but the fact is, that trials at several different times, made by adding a solution of acetate of lead, only gave a white precipitate ; shewing therefore the absence of this gas, unless in the most inconsiderable proportion.

*Analysis.*

In a pint,                                            Grains.

    Muriate of soda..........22·60
    Muriate of lime......... 3·68
    ————— magnesia ..... 5·16
    Sulphate of soda........52·32

              83·76

Oxide of iron, a minute portion.

## No. 3.

Described as *magnesian saline.*
Taste, saline and chalybeate.
Specific gravity, 1·0083.

The action of tests produces the same effects as with the preceding waters, with the important exception that the tincture of galls produced a purple hue mixed with brown, distinctly indicating the presence of iron ; and prussiate of potash a considerable shade of green, with a precipitate.

*Analysis.*

In a pint,

Grains.

| | |
|---|---|
| Muriate of soda | 17·60 |
| Muriate of lime | 3·08 |
| ——— magnesia | 3·30 |
| Sulphate of soda | 43·20 |

67·18

Oxide of iron, probably a grain in a gallon.

## No. 4.

Described as *pure saline.*
Taste, strongly saline.
Specific gravity, 1·0122.

The tests act as before described in respect to the saline ingredients, but scarcely afford any evidence of the presence of iron.

*Analysis.*

In a pint,

| | Grains. |
|---|---|
| Muriate of soda........... | 47·80 |
| ——— lime.......... | 4·29 |
| ——— magnesia...... | 7·30 |
| Sulphate of soda.......... | 59 20 |
| | 118·59 |

Oxide of iron, a trace.

A review of the composition of these waters points out that the number called strong aerated chalybeate, cannot be entitled to such an appellation. Its carbonic acid is insufficient to redden litmus paper distinctly; its iron almost fails to affect the prussiate of potash, and produces only a slight change of colour with the tincture of galls. It may be pronounced to be a very good saline alterative water, and slightly chalybeate.

No. 2, very feebly indeed answers to the name of sulphureous. I learn that this and the other sulphuretted waters at Cheltenham communicate to characters written on paper with acetate of lead, a discolouration after some hours, the paper being fixed to the trap door; but the fresh waters, all, produce with acetate of lead a white precipitate\*.

No. 3, which is commonly called magnesian saline, is in fact almost as strongly impreg-

---

\* I found that Harrogate water, which had been kept three or four months, diluted with fifteen parts of distilled water, gave, with acetate of lead, a brown hue, quite characteristic.

nated with iron as any water in Cheltenham. Its saline impregnation is not strong, but it deserves to be esteemed as a water considerably chalybeate, and mildly saline.

No. 4 appears from the analysis to be the most active of the saline waters. Making a course of experiments with two specimens of this water sent to me within a short interval, I was surprised by the difference of result, and after a strict inquiry into the cause, I found that the proprietor was in the habit of adding a concentrated solution of the evaporated salts to this water; and hence the obvious explanation of its varying composition.

### THOMPSON'S WELLS, OR MONTPELIER SPA.

I have already mentioned that the original spa became in use about the year 1718. The following particulars of Mr. Thompson's Wells, I take the liberty of quoting from the analysis published by W. T. Brande, Esq. and Samuel Parkes, Esq.; and to which I shall afterwards refer as the analysis of 1817.

" For many years subsequent to this period, the properties of these waters * were treated of by various medical writers; and between the years 1770 and 1780 they acquired so much reputation, that the town became a place of great resort for invalids, from all parts of the kingdom.

---

* Viz. of the Original Spa.

" But as the celebrity of the waters increased, it was soon found that the wells could not supply the quantity which was required by the increased demand ; and in the year 1788 a new well was sunk by order of his late Majesty (George III.), known by the name of the *King's Well*.   At first the supply from this well was very abundant; but it afterwards decreased so much, that it was often drank out by the company in half an hour.

" The waters of all the wells having thus continued to diminish in quantity, serious apprehensions were entertained that the company, which had been in the habit of visiting Cheltenham, would meet with such frequent disappointments from the failure of the springs, that they would be induced to look out for some other watering place, and in a short time the town would be entirely deserted by the strangers who had formerly visited it, either for the purposes of health or pleasure.

" At this period (1806) a gentleman of the name of Thompson, who had purchased a great part of the land in the vicinity of Cheltenham, determined to search for mineral water on his own estate, and to try to supply the deficiency so much complained of.   The success he met with soon led him to think of turning this discovery to his own advantage, as well as that of the public; and accordingly a new pump-room was erected, and no exertions were spared, until water was obtained sufficient for the supply of whatever company might resort to the town and neighbourhood."

## No. 1.

Described by the proprietor as the *strong chalybeate saline water.* Depth of well 45 feet.

Taste, saline and slightly bitter.

Specific gravity, 1·0085.

The action of tests both with this and the remaining waters at this spa, act in the manner described with Old Well, No. 1, in regard to the saline ingredients, varying only in degree according to the relative strength of the impregnation.

A faint indication of the presence of iron is produced by tincture of galls.

Prussiate of potash occasions a very slight green tinge.

### *Analysis.*

In a pint,

| | Grains. |
|---|---|
| Muriate of soda | 55·50 |
| —————— lime | 3·31 |
| —————— magnesia | 2·10 |
| Sulphate of soda | 21·80 |
| | 82·71 |

Oxide of iron, a minute portion.

The following statement appears in the analysis of 1817.

" The specific gravity, 1·0092*.

" One wine pint contains **74** grains of dry salts (after having been kept for six hours at a temperature of **212°**) consisting of

Grains.

| | |
|---|---|
| Muriate of soda | 41·3 |
| Sulphate of soda | 22·7 |
| Sulphate of magnesia | 6·0 |
| Sulphate of lime | 2·5 |
| Carbonate of soda and iron | 1·5 |
| | **74·0** |

" In a pint about **2·5** cubic inches of carbonic acid."

## No. 2.

Described as the strong *sulphuretted saline water*. Depth of well 48 feet. The pipe goes to the bottom.

Taste, chiefly saline.

Specific gravity, 1·0065.

Tincture of galls produces an effect just distinguishable, indicating the presence of iron.

Prussiate of potash, the very slightest shade of green.

Acetate of lead, a white precipitate.

---

* After the loss of the gaseous contents. The same circumstance is mentioned in the examination of the other waters.

*Analysis.*

In a pint,

Grains.

Muriate of soda........... 25·70

———— lime........... 3·31

———— magnesia....... 1·52

Sulphate of soda .......... 21·76

———————

52·29

Oxide of iron, a minute portion.

According to the analysis of 1817.

" Specific gravity, 1·0085.

" In a pint,

Grains.

Muriate of soda........... 35

Sulphate of soda.......... 23·5

Sulphate of magnesia........ 5·0

Sulphate of lime........... 1·2

Oxide of iron............. ·3

———————

65·0

" Gaseous contents.

Cubic inches.

Sulphuretted hydrogen ....... 2.5

Carbonic acid .............. 1·5

———————

4·0"

## No. 3.

Described as the weak *sulphuretted saline water*. Same well as No. 2. The pipe goes to within two feet of the bottom of the well.

Taste, saline and mildly chalybeate.

Specific gravity, 1·0067.

The tincture of galls produces a very light brown; the prussiate of potash just a shade of green.

### *Analysis.*

In a pint,

|  | Grains. |
|---|---|
| Muriate of soda | 31·00 |
| —————— lime | 1·84 |
| —————— magnesia | 2·05 |
| Sulphate of soda | 22·80 |
|  | 57·69 |

Oxide of iron, a trace.

According to the analysis of 1817.

" Specific gravity, 1·006.

" In a pint,

|  | Grains. |
|---|---|
| Muriate of soda | 15·0 |
| Sulphate of soda | 14·0 |
| Sulphate of magnesia | 5·0 |
| Sulphate of lime | 1·5 |
| Oxide of iron | ·5 |
|  | 36·0 |

" Gaseous contents.

|  | Cubic Inches. |
|---|---|
| Sulphuretted hydrogen | 2·5 |
| Carbonic acid | 1·5 |
|  | 4·0" |

## No. 4.

Described as the *pure saline water*. Depth of well, 50 feet.

Taste, pleasantly saline.

Specific gravity, 1·0077.

Neither tincture of galls nor prussiate of potash produce any apparent change.

### *Analysis.*

In a pint,

Grains.

| | |
|---|---|
| Muriate of soda........ ....... | 46·40 |
| ———— lime.......... | 3·07 |
| ———— magnesia....... | 2·02 |
| Sulphate of soda.......... | 28·64 |

80·13

According to the analysis of 1817.

" Specific gravity, 1·010.

" In a pint,

Grains.

| | |
|---|---|
| Muriate of soda...... ..... | 50·0 |
| Sulphate of soda........... | 15·0 |
| Sulphate of magnesia....... | 11·0 |
| Sulphate of lime........... | 4·5 |

80·5

## No. 5.

Described as the *sulphuretted and chalybeated magnesian spring, or bitter saline water*. Depth of well 60 feet.

Taste, saline and rather bitter.

Specific gravity, 1·0065.

Acetate of lead produces a white precipitate.

Tincture of galls affords a very faint indication of the presence of iron.

Prussiate of potash produces a very slight shade of green.

*Analysis.*

In a pint,

Grains.

| | |
|---|---|
| Muriate of soda | 23·50 |
| ————— lime | 4·92 |
| ————— magnesia | 3·61 |
| Sulphate of soda | 38·80 |

70·83

Oxide of iron a minute portion.

According to the analysis of 1817.

" Specific gravity, 1.008.

" In a pint,

Grains.

| | |
|---|---|
| Sulphate of magnesia | 36·5 |
| Muriate of magnesia | 9·0 |
| Muriate of soda | 9·5 |
| Sulphate of lime | 3·5 |
| Oxide of iron | 3·5 |
| Loss | 1·0 |

63·0"

No. 6.

Described as the *saline chalybeate,* drawn from the well near the laboratory ; depth of which is 126 feet.

Taste, saline and slightly bitter.

Specific gravity, 1·0098.

Tincture of galls produces a faint appearance of the presence of iron.

Prussiate of potash, a shade of green a little more marked than No. 5.

*Analysis.*

In a pint,

| | Grains. |
|---|---|
| Muriate of soda | 76·15 |
| —————— lime | 3·07 |
| —————— magnesia | 3·02 |
| Sulphate of soda | 11·62 |
| | 93·86 |

Oxide of iron, a minute portion.

Gaseous contents.

According to the analysis of 1817.

" Specific gravity, 1·004.

" In a pint,

| | Grains. |
|---|---|
| Muriate of soda | 22·0 |
| Sulphate of soda | 10·0 |
| Oxide of iron | 1·5 |
| Loss | 0·5 |
| | 34·0." |

Carbonic acid, about 10 cubic inches.

It is evident from the comparative view of these analyses, that the waters in the course of the last few years have undergone considerable changes ; and these changes apply particularly to Nos. 1, 2, 3, 5. No. 1 now scarcely contains any chalybeate impregnation ;—I am persuaded,

not half a grain of iron in a gallon.    The No. 2
no longer claims to be called a strong sulphuretted water, nor No. 3 even weakly impregnated
with the gas.    The analysis of 1817 represents
No. 2 to be even more strongly impregnated
than the powerful water of Harrogate (see p.
98) ; but now it produces only a white precipitate
with the acetate of lead.    No. 5, which is described to have contained the immense proportion of 3·5 grs. of oxide of iron in a pint, now is
only affected in a slight degree either by the tincture of galls, or the prussiate of potash.

I am compelled therefore to give the following character of these waters.    No. 1, a saline
aperient alterative water, containing a very slight
impregnation of iron, so as not to be objectionable on this account, except with a patient to
whom this ingredient is forbidden even in a
small quantity.

No. 2, of much the same power as No 1, except that it has less of the muriates of soda and
magnesia.    It does not appear to be more
strongly chalybeate than No. 1.

No. 3, equally aperient with No. 2 ; has less
of muriate of lime, and more of muriate of magnesia.

No. 4 is a saline water, which appears to be
wholly free from iron, but contains a good proportion of all the saline ingredients.

No. 5 is a water not shewing any sulphuretted

impregnation. It is only slightly chalybeate. It possesses a fuller impregnation both of aperient salt, and of the most important muriates, than the other waters.

No. 6 contains only a minute proportion of iron. It is less aperient than No. 4, but contains rather more muriate of magnesia.

### THE SHERBORNE SPA.

These wells are situated at the top of the long walk from the Colonnade in the High Street, between Thompson's Spa and the Old Well, and are connected with a spacious and elegant pump room.

The pumps are in number four. In regard to their saline ingredients the action of tests is precisely of the same nature with that produced on the preceding waters, the effects varying only in degree.

The water described as *sulphureous and chalybeate.*

Taste, saline and slightly chalybeate.

Specific gravity, 1·0011.

The action of tests demonstrates that this water is one of slight impregnation. This is obvious also from its low specific gravity.

Tincture of galls quickly produces a light purple colour.

Prussiate of potash, a slight shade of green.

Acetate of lead produces a white precipitate.

*Analysis.*

In a pint,

|  | Grains. |
|---|---|
| Muriate of soda............. | 3 31 |
| ——— of lime............. | 1·23 |
| ——— magnesia ........a trace | |
| Sulphate of soda............ | 4·37 |
| | 8·91 |

Oxide of iron, probably half a grain in
a gallon.

The water described as *pure saline.*

Taste, saline.

Specific gravity, 1·009.

Neither tincture of galls nor prussiate of potash produce any indication of the presence of iron in this water.

*Analysis.*

In a pint,

|  | Grains. |
|---|---|
| Muriate of soda........72·8 | |
| ——— lime ......... | 4·29 |
| ——— magnesia...... | ·59 |
| Sulphate of soda........ | 6·76 |
| | 84·44 |

The water described as the *magnesian* water.

Taste, almost negative.

Specific gravity 1·0012.

Tincture of galls produces a light brown colour ; prussiate of potash, a pale grass green. All the other tests act but slightly.

*Analysis.*

In a pint,

Grains.

Muriate of soda.........1·67

——————— lime........1·85

——————— magnesia, a trace.

Sulphate of soda........2·43

—————

5·95

### No. 4*.

It appears that this water is in reality the pure saline, but is denominated No. 4, by way of making a correspondence in numbers with the waters of the other wells. The close agreement which I found in the specific gravity, action of tests, and results of analysis, between this water and the pure saline, renders it unnecessary for me to enter into further particulars respecting it.

In giving a summary view of the waters of this spa, I am led to describe the first, as a mild chalybeate, and light alterative saline. I consider that the oxide of iron can scarcely exceed half a grain in a gallon.

I must here notice, that the saline contents of the Cheltenham waters materially influence the

—————————————————

* This is the only water numbered at this Spa.

action of tincture of galls and prussiate of potash, as I discovered by a series of comparative experiments with a solution of sulphate of iron mixed with Cheltenham water after it had deposited its iron, and with distilled water. The tincture of galls produces shades of brown with the saline water, instead of purple; prussiate of potash, shades of verdegris green, instead of blue. If the impregnation with iron be weak, the change produced by the prussiate takes place very slowly. In these experiments, I obtained further information of the proportions of iron indicated by the particular action of the tests; and hence my deductions of the probable quantity of iron in these, and the waters of Leamington which are to follow.

The second water contains a good share of the muriate of lime; but, from its small proportion of sulphate of soda, is but very slightly aperient. It must be considered therefore chiefly as a saline alterative water.

The third is improperly called magnesian water, which would imply a strong impregnation with magnesia. It is altogether a very weak water.

In taking a general review of the composition of all these waters, we find that there are three kinds, all saline, aperient, and alterative; some containing also a very feeble sulphuretted impregnation; others a small portion of oxide of iron held in solution by carbonic acid.

When I observe that by the term aperient I

designate the sulphate of soda as the ingredient; and by the term alterative, the muriates of lime and magnesia ; the reader can readily draw a comparison between the relative strength of the different waters.

It is the practice to increase the purgative power of Thompson's No. 4, by the addition of a solution of the salts obtained by evaporation of the water. I made a series of experiments with this solution, and found it to consist of about three parts of sulphate of soda, one part of sulphate of magnesia, and a portion of muriate of soda. It was not affected by oxalate of ammonia; it did not, therefore, contain lime. I must here beg to suggest an improvement on the method of increasing the power of the water, and recommend that No. 4, for example, should be concentrated by evaporation, to about half, and offered to the drinker as strong No. 4. In this case it will be increased in the strength of its muriates, which does not happen by the present method; for the muriates of lime and magnesia being very deliquescent, become removed from the evaporated dry mass. If the water thus strengthened do not prove sufficiently aperient, its action should be assisted by some suitable pills taken at bed time. No. 2 of the Old Well is almost a pure saline, which may be treated in the same manner, but being a stronger natural water than Thompson's No. 4, it need not be concentrated to more than a third.

I call this pure saline, for I have not discovered it to possess any sulphuretted impregnation which need be regarded ; but as I am persuaded the waters vary in regard to the proportion of sulphuretted hydrogen gas, I would say, that if any particular water should, by its taste and smell, discover itself to be so impregnated, and on that account be objectionable, Thompson's No. 4 will deserve the preference. The strongest of the Sherborne waters is more of a saline alterative than saline aperient.

I have a few remarks to offer on the salts prepared at Mr. Thompson's laboratory, and upon what is called in a note in the Analysis of 1817, " a murio-sulphate of magnesia and iron in brown crystals, highly tonic."

The saline preparations are termed

1. Crystallized alkaline sulphates ; or crystals of real Cheltenham salts.

2. Ditto effloresced and ground to an impalpable powder for hot climates.

3. Magnesian sulphate, in a state of efflorescence.

The crystalline salt 1 appears to consist almost wholly of sulphate of soda ; but it also contains a small portion of magnesia, which, from the deliquescence of the salt, we may consider to be combined with muriatic acid. It probably also contains a little muriate of soda.

o

The effloresced salt 11 is, as already descr bed, the crystallized salt 1 ground to powder.

The magnesian sulphate 3, is composed of sulphate of soda and sulphate of magnesia, but of the former salt in much the larger proportion.

The murio-sulphate of magnesia and iron, consists chiefly of sulphate of magnesia, a small portion of muriate of magnesia, and a little oxide of iron attached to it mechanically, having fallen down from its solvent the carbonic acid, which is dissipated in the process of evaporation. This salt, upon being dissolved in water, parts with its adhering oxide of iron which is wholly insoluble in water. The fluid is not in the least degree affected by tincture of galls, however much it may be concentrated*.

From the foregoing premises, the conclusion follows, that a patient does not pursue a course of the Cheltenham waters by merely taking the dissolved salts, for he loses those valuable ingredients the muriates of lime and magnesia, and loses the chalybeate principle, which, however weak in these waters, must be allowed a considerable share of useful action. The true character,

---

* Since making my examination of these salts, my attention has been directed to Mr. Phillips's paper on the same subject, in Thompson's Annals of Philosophy, vol ii. This Chemist arrived at the same general results. I refer the reader to his more elaborate account.

195

therefore, of the Cheltenham salts is now made sufficiently apparent to render further comment unnecessary.

---

## MEDICAL HISTORY.

BEFORE I enter upon the medicinal employment of the Cheltenham waters, I find it necessary to give a slight further discussion of their chemical properties. The method of analysis did not allow of our obtaining the carbonates; but we found by an experiment of slowly boiling one of the waters, which contained the largest quantity of muriate of lime, that a very trivial portion only of carbonate of lime fell down. In the computation of the ingredients according to Murray's view, it is necessary to consider that the sulphuric acid is altogether combined with the soda, as forming the most soluble salt, and consequently that all the magnesia is combined with muriatic acid. No sulphate of magnesia, therefore, in this view of the subject, can be obtained except in the direct method of analysis, and as the result of decomposition of the salts, during the process of evaporation.

It is incumbent on me to take some notice of a pamphlet recently published by Dr. Adam Neale on the Cheltenham waters, in which he endeavours to extol the character of the water of

o 2

the Old Well, at the expence of the waters of the Montpelier Spa. Wishing to avoid all controversy, except as I may be led into it for the sake of science and truth, I shall not express a conjecture as to the motives which could dictate the publication of these pages ; but I must observe, that the author would have consulted his own reputation ; the consideration fairly due to the proprietor of the Montpelier Spa ; the welfare of the town of Cheltenham ; and I may add, even the cause of humanity ; if, before he had made public such statements as he has given, he had informed himself of their truth. The bases of his opinions being founded in a want of sufficient acquaintance with the chemical composition of the waters, his reflections cannot be entitled to serious regard ; nor can the medical character of the waters possibly sustain any permanent injury from his satirical aspersion. It is true that he has deduced his conclusions from the analyses made by others, and, therefore, so far has a colourable support for his opinions. But, I must remark, the analysis of the water of the Old Well, from which he draws his comparison, was made by Dr. Fothergill so far back as the year 1788, a distant period when the true processes of analytical chemistry were but little understood. Also when the Analysis of 1817 was published, Dr. Murray had not made known his ingenious views on the subject, and which appear so worthy to be adopted. Dr. Neale has placed in parallel columns the following tabular view, exhibiting the analysis of the Old Well, No. 1, by Dr. Fothergill, and No. 1 of Montpelier Spa, by Messrs. Brande and Parkes.

### Original Spa Water,
One pint,

|  | Grains. |
|---|---|
| Sulphate of soda........ }<br>Sulphate of magnesia } | 60·0 |
| Iron ........................... | ·6 |
| Muriate of soda.............. | ·6 |
| Sulphate of lime............ | 5·0 |
| Carbon. & muriate of }<br>magnesia.............. } | 3·1 |
|  | 69·3 |

GASEOUS CONTENTS.

|  | Cubic Inches. |
|---|---|
| Carbonic acid............... | 3·7 |
| Sulphuretted hydrogen... | 1·8 |
|  | 5·5 |

### Montpelier Spa, No. 1.
One pint,

|  | Grains. |
|---|---|
| Sulphate of soda 22·7 }<br>Sulph. of magnesia 6·0 } | 28·7 |
| Soda and iron carbonates | 1·5 |
| Muriate of soda............ | 41·3 |
| Sulphate of lime........... | 2·5 |
|  | 74·0 |

GASEOUS CONTENTS.

|  | Cubic Inches. |
|---|---|
| Carbonic acid............... | 2·5 |

In opposition to this comparative view, I shall report the following, as derived from my present analysis:

### Original Spa, No. 1.
In a pint,

|  | Grains. |
|---|---|
| Muriate of soda......... | 58·20 |
| Muriate of lime......... | 6·21 |
| ———— magnesia ... | 2·54 |
| Sulphate of soda........ | 14·56 |
|  | 81·51 |

A slight indication of iron.

### Montpelier, No. 1.
In a pint,

|  | Grains. |
|---|---|
| Muriate of soda......... | 55·50 |
| Muriate of lime......... | 3·31 |
| ———— magnesia... | 2·10 |
| Sulphate of soda........ | 21·80 |
|  | 82·71 |

A slight indication of iron.

From these tables it appears, that the water, No. 1, of the Old Well, contains a larger proportion of the muriate of lime, than any of the other waters ; and therefore, as respects this ingredient, it is the most alterative. The point, however, insisted upon by Dr. Neale, is perfectly without foundation. He offers an opinion, which appears to me infinitely over-charged, if not altogether fanciful, of the hazardous stimulating properties of the muriate of soda. He condemns the Montpelier water as containing this injurious excess of muriate of soda, and an inferior proportion of aperient salt, as compared with the other water : The very contrary now appears. He censures in harsh terms the custom of adding an artificial solution of salts to the natural water. But it should be observed, that it is only done when the drinker desires. I have shewn that this custom has equally prevailed (although unknown) at the Old Well, with the No 4; and I have suggested a mode which I think preferable. He argues that the invalid visitor might derive great benefit from taking a solution of Epsom and Glauber salts, at home, observing all the rules, as by drinking the Cheltenham water with such added solution. He seems to have no idea that the composition of these waters is to be esteemed important, not merely as containing ingredients of an aperient nature, but as being truly alterative ; or, in other words, possessing powers which operate medicinally in a gradual

manner, not affecting the patient very sensibly
at the time, but tending from day to day to alter
and improve the functions of the digestive organs ;
and consequently to change the condition of the
whole system. If we take, for example, a water,
as No. 1 of either of these wells, containing the
oxide of iron held in solution by carbonic acid
in conjunction with the several saline ingredients,
we have a composition not easily imitable by art.
The influence of a small portion of oxide of iron
in a water, must not be estimated exactly by its
quantity, as is so well shewn by the power of the
Bath water when used fresh from the pump.

I shall be happy if my observations may tend
to redeem the Cheltenham waters from the unjust
reflections so lately thrown upon them. Nature
is not in error. She presents her excellent springs
with a liberal hand, and with full claims upon
the confidence of the invalid. If hitherto the
best management have not been exercised in the
plan of adding to the strength of the waters, I
doubt not that the proprietors will gladly put in
practice any improvement which may be suggested.

I now gladly retire from this unpleasant discussion, to which I have been impelled by the
nature of my inquiry, and by a sense of justice
which I have felt to be due to the occasion.

The medical character of the waters may be

comprised within a brief sketch, after the dissertation already given on their composition.

I consider the point fairly established, that the
nature of the Cheltenham waters as a medicine, is
not to be considered as simply a saline aperient in
a diluent form.   Happily for society, the real
merits of any remedy do not depend upon the
caprice of individual opinion, upon ignorance, or
upon the fluctuations of fashion and prejudice.
The Cheltenham waters have established for themselves a high character because they have de-
served it.   This important effect belongs to them ;
—that an invalid can pursue a continued daily
course, such as produces a regular and considerable action on the bowels, without suffering that
debility of the constitution and impaired appetite,
which are apt to occur from a similar course of
saline aperients at home.   Witness the keen
relish with which the breakfast meal is eaten,
after the early visit to the wells : And the general
improvement of health and spirits consequent to
the judicious use of the waters, is as remarkable
as it is important.

It is a very common error of invalids to think
that the Cheltenham waters are a very simple remedy ; from which cause they do not allow themselves
to consider that any previous medical advice is necessary.   I affirm, without fear of contradiction,
that much harm continually arises from this ill-

judged confidence ; and I have had the opportu-
nities of observing how much some patients have
injured themselves by not taking the waters upon
a proper plan, and by continuing them for an improper period. As a general rule, a mercurial
purgative should precede the use of the water. It
is an important fact, that if much confinement of
the bowels have prevailed, and more especially if
there be decided biliary obstruction, the water, instead of becoming the ready remedy which is expected, may prove a source of evil in the way I shall
state. It may act upon the exhalant vessels of
the alimentary canal, so as to produce only fluid
discharge, and actually leave behind the more
solid and obstructing matter. The same observation applies in a great degree to the use of the water
in progress. It is, I know, the medical practice at
Cheltenham. and very judiciously, to conjoin the
use of a purgative alterative pill with the water.
This will of course be more or less active in its
composition, according to the constitution of the
patient and the nature of the case. The patient
being fitly prepared, has next to be instructed as
to his choice in the No. of the water. It will
generally happen that at first he should commence
with a purely saline water, the dose of which will
obviously be regulated by the effect which is
desired to be produced. It happens with some
persons of peculiar constitution, that the water
does not pass off by the bowels, but chiefly re-

mains in the canal, causing a distressing degree
of distension.  Now, in this case I do not advise
that the use of the water be abandoned; but if,
notwithstanding the auxiliary action of pills, it
thus disagree, let the patient take the concentrated water as described, p. 192, in a smaller
quantity; for example, a quarter of a pint as
a dose, employing it only as an alterative,
and looking entirely to the influence of medicine
for the action of the bowels.  Hence, it will
probably act well on the kidnies, and as a very
useful alterative in improving the digestive
organs.

The water being used upon this principle, an
active or an immediate good effect is not to be
expected.  The patient must have patience.  I
approve very much of the custom of giving a
little increase in temperature to the water.  When
the proper moment arrives for changing the
pure saline for one of the chalybeate waters, the
same general principles are to be kept in view,
in regard to the management of the bowels.  It
is obvious, that as sulphuretted waters, the
Cheltenham springs are not entitled to much
consideration.  Some persons are so exquisitely
sensible to the influence of chalybeate medicines,
that they cannot with any precautions make use
of a water containing even a minute portion of
iron.  Such individuals therefore must confine
themselves to the pure saline; but the majority

of patients will derive material advantage, from having the tonic influence of the iron added to the other properties of the water.

I shall now give a concise account of the principal disorders, in which, the Cheltenham waters are particularly applicable.

The gouty patient may drink the pure saline waters of Cheltenham, with almost certain prospect of advantage. He must be prepared for the course, and I wish, once for all, to extend this injunction of *proper preparation* to every patient in every case. It very commonly happens that in a short time after commencing the water, a paroxysm of gout takes place. Whence does this arise?—Not, in my opinion, from the aperient qualities of the water—nor from its gaseous impregnation, which is not active; but from the stimulating qualities of the muriates. Under these circumstances I would wish a discontinuance of the water during the active symptoms of gout, which might be treated on the principles recommended in my Treatise, if receiving the approbation of the attendant physician; and, when the convalescence begins, the water is to be resumed. I believe I am warranted in saying, that in all probability a fit of gout produced by the Cheltenham water will not soon be followed by another attack; provided also that the case has been in every respect well managed, and the patient has taken due prophylactic care.

The disordered conditions of the digestive organs, which comprehend the several kinds of dyspepsia, hepatic obstruction, and torpor of the bowels, rank foremost in the class of Cheltenham cases. The East Indian visits these springs almost as a matter of course, upon his arrival in this country.

The value of the Cheltenham waters, as a remedy in dyspepsia, will depend entirely on the nature of the case. If real and primary debility of stomach be the cause, the waters are not forbidden, but must be taken with much circumspection ; and rather as an alterative than an active aperient. A spring affording the chalybeate principle will soon deserve the preference, if not in the first instance. If dyspepsia arise, as it often does, from a course of repletion ;—from frequently repeated over excitement, the water may be taken freely without apprehension ; and for the most part, the pure saline will be the kind of water most appropriate.

The jaundiced patient will require more preparation, and more particular attention in the combined use of medicines, than any other description of invalid.

It would be incompatible with my present purpose to enter into any extended consideration of the nature and treatment of hepatic complaint. It is an encouraging consideration, for those who labour under disordered functions of the liver, together with debility of the constitution, that the action of the Cheltenham water on the bowels, from day to day, is not attended with the weakening effect which is liable to happen from ordinary medicine; and as the individual who has resided in a tropical climate, most usually has undermined the real powers of his constitution, this is a point of great moment.

Every practitioner must have met with cases of diseased liver, accompanied with such an impaired state of constitution, that any active employment of mercury would be an unwise if not a hazardous treatment. It is not safe to raise up mercurial fever in the system in these instances; and I do not believe that a better expedient can be adopted, than a course of Cheltenham saline water in conjunction with a mild mercurial alterative.

The term *bilious* is certainly of late years so general a phrase, that it becomes an expression adopted in every disordered state of stomach, and is applied to every state of the liver, whether it be torpid in its action and fail to furnish bile, or be in a state of irritation, secreting in excess. If the erroneous view first described be taken, it probably happens that calomel is resorted to imprudently and without occasion. A patient is a very bad judge upon these points of discrimination.

It happens, as an occasional inconvenience,

from the Cheltenham waters, that irritation is excited in the mucous membrane of the lower intestines, and painful hemorrhoids are produced. I have known even a degree of dysentery to take place. I think it will be found, for the most part, in these cases, that a predisposition to such forms of complaint has existed, and that the action of the water merely proves the exciting cause. Should such complaints arise, it is obvious that the use of the water should be suspended, and that the inconveniences in question should receive exclusive attention. In gravel, a course of the water, in union with alterative medicine, is much to be recommended.

Those who are subject to erysipelas, erythema, urticaria, and the different forms of acne, will most probably derive advantage from a course of the pure saline Cheltenham water, joining with it some alterative medicine. The cutaneous diseases, mentioned at p. 105, claim rather the use of Harrogate water, as already explained.

The addition of the warm bath, upon a regular plan, will be material in assisting the alterative action of the water. It should be used so as not to prove a considerable relaxant; and it is indeed desirable that it should produce the opposite effect, and be made auxiliary to the general tone of the system.

With such a view, the patient should bathe an hour or two before dinner, and not take any unnecessary exercise after it. The temperature of the confined warm bath, should not be less than 93° nor more than 95°; but the uniform temperature should be attentively kept up. Not less than ten minutes, and not more than twenty, may be expressed as a good general rule for the duration of the immersion; and from once to three times in the week, as to frequency.

At Mr. Thompson's baths, there is one* so conveniently spacious that the patient can keep in free motion the whole time, and the temperature of the water may be regulated from 80° to 100°, with a little care on the part of attendants. So considerable a body of water cannot very well be maintained at an uniform temperature; but much may be done in this respect; and it appears to me that this large bath may, in many cases, be infinitely serviceable.

If, with the best management, the general immersion in the warm bath prove too relaxing to the constitution, the shower bath used upon a principle of graduation as to the temperature and quantity of the water, will deserve a trial. It is an important remedy, and, when judiciously managed, scarcely ever fails to agree perfectly and prove very useful.

---

* I learn that its admeasurement is 12 feet by 10. I believe that every kind of bath is obtained at Cheltenham in great perfection.

The diet of the invalid at a watering place should be studiously moderate and correct. This is a point of peculiar moment when the patient is under a course of these waters. The quantity of fluid at all the meals should be much restricted; for otherwise the muscular power of the stomach and intestinal canal may become weakened from distension. Half-a-pint of aqueous fluid with the dinner meal is amply sufficient. Soda water, or plain water, made palatable with toast, or any other simple addition, should be the exclusive beverage, with the exception of such moderate quantity of good wine as may be allowed. Soups, unless plain gravy soup, and that sparingly, should be avoided. As a general rule, I should class in the prohibited list, salt meat, pork, fat and skin of meat, rich made dishes, the fat part of salmon, stewed eels, lobsters, pickles, and salads; spinage, as being a vegetable which readily ferments; any vegetable which is not quite in season, sweet, tender, and well boiled; pie crust, and all rich confectionary; strong cheese, and such as is either very new or very old. These are my brief directions as to the quality of the food, but the quantity is also a most cardinal point of attention. What reasonable expectation of benefit can be entertained from a course of alterative aperient waters, if a system of repletion with various kinds of stimulating food be every day pursued? The liberal

regime of a boarding house is in this respect unfavourable to the necessary discipline of the patient; but it is incumbent on him to exercise a
virtuous forbearance. Meat should be eaten only
once a day, unless in the instance of a delicacy
of constitution. A new laid egg lightly boiled
at breakfast, and biscuits in the middle of the
day; will sufficiently support the stomach till the
dinner hour, which should not be later than five.
White fish, and boiled rather than fried, is the
most wholesome. I must observe, that where
strict regimen is necessary, salmon must be forbidden. One kind of meat only should be eaten,
and if poultry or game be added, the quantity
should be small. Game should not be eaten
when high: It is then too stimulating. Game is
too often rendered improper for the stomach of
the invalid, by the rich sauces with which it is
dressed. In young game every part is tender;
when old, the very muscular parts should be
avoided. With regard to meats, when the animal is not too aged, it is the muscular fibre which
affords the best stimulus to the stomach, and is
the most easy of digestion. Mutton and beef seem
to be most digestible when roasted; veal, when
boiled.* This last may be stated to be the least

---

* I conceive that the skin and cellular part of meat are
more favourably prepared for the agency of the gastric juice
(to speak familiarly, are rendered more easy of digestion) by

P

digestible of the meats in general; and the fact appears referable to a principle which I think may be laid down, that animals which are allowed to range in fields, acquire much muscle and little fat in proportion, while the reverse of this takes place in the stall-fed cattle, which become much covered with cellular texture and fat.

I consider it a good rule to eat only one kind of vegetable at the same meal. In regard to dessert, the least quantity is the best, and I would forbid raw apples and pears, plums of every kind, gooseberries and currants, and melon. I repeat that these restrictions apply to the individual who visits Cheltenham really on account of health. Those who drink the waters from accident rather than by prescription, may abide by these good rules or not, at choice. It will often be a valuable part of the plan of drinking the Cheltenham waters, to suspend the course after about three weeks; then to go to Malvern for a week or ten days, and upon its health-inspiring hills gain increase of tone in the constitution; when, with

---

the influence of the boiling process; but, on the contrary, that muscular parts are rendered comparatively more loose in their texture by means of roasting. As illustrations of the probability of this reasoning, I may mention the articles calf's foot and veal, to exemplify the first position; and the second is instanced by the superior tenderness of beef moderately roasted, over that which has long been submitted to the boiling temperature.

double advantage, another fortnight may be devoted to the waters ; resumed, however, rather as alteratives than active aperients.

In that very necessary part of regimen, regular daily exercise, the patient should be careful to avoid exposure, and indeed all active exertion, during the mid-day sun. In summer, the heat at Cheltenham is very considerable; and the invalid must be careful, by all good management, to preserve the powers of his constitution, in order to do full justice to a course of the waters.

I have to conclude with a short account of the pure chalybeate waters of Cheltenham.

### FOWLER'S OR CAMBRAY CHALYBEATE.

The water is transparent, not sparkling, and to the taste moderately chalybeate.

Its specific gravity is 1·0011.

### ACTION OF TESTS.

Neither litmus nor hyacinth paper undergo any change of colour.

Tincture of galls almost immediately produces a slight purple.

Prussiate of potash, after a few minutes, produces a faint blue tint.

P 2

With the boiled water, no change of colour is occasioned by these re-agents.

Nitrate of silver, a considerable precipitate.

Carbonate of ammonia and phosphate of soda, applied in succession, produce the compound precipitate of lime and the triple phosphate of magnesia, as formerly described.

Pure ammonia renders the water slightly milky.

Muriate of barytes produces a dense cloud.

Oxalate of ammonia a similar effect.

From the low specific gravity of this water, we may conclude that it is not strongly impregnated ; and from the action of the tests we are entitled to infer that it contains lime and magnesia, with sulphuric and muriatic acids, and oxide of iron held in solution by carbonic acid.

BARRATT'S CHALYBEATE.

The specific gravity of this water is 1·001

ACTION OF TESTS.

Tincture of galls does not produce any immediate change of colour, and, after standing, the tint of purple is only faint.

Prussiate of potash produces a very slight effect, and that slowly.

All the other re-agents act in the same manner as with Fowler's chalybeate, but in a less degree.

Hence we may certainly conclude, that this water is precisely of the same character as Fowler's, but in all respects weaker.

In regard to the medical report of these chalybeate waters, I need only refer the reader to my Observations on the Tunbridge Wells Water. The Cambray spring evidently deserves the preference. An invalid having concluded a course of the saline aperient waters, if making a longer stay at Cheltenham, may, with advantage, have recourse to this mild pure chalybeate, and which contains also some useful saline ingredients. It is due, however, to Tunbridge Wells, to say, that as a pure carbonated chalybeate, its springs rank the first ; and deservedly enjoy a higher reputation than any other water of the same kind in this country.

# LEAMINGTON.

LEAMINGTON, or, as sometimes called, Leamington Priors, is situated two miles east of Warwick ; and distant from London 90 miles. Its name is derived from the Leam, a small stream, which passes near it; and the term Priors refers to the monastery of Kenilworth, to which it was formerly attached. It may be further described as situated at the eastern side of that extensive flat, called the Plain of Warwick, and which is covered with the formation called, in this country, the red marl. This bed is the same as that in which the salt mines in Cheshire are placed, and it also frequently contains gypsum. Accordingly both these minerals are found at Leamington : the salt however is not met with in the state of rock, but only as a salt spring. To the east lies the lias, and the oolite range.

A stronger example of the prosperous influence upon a place, derived from its fortunate possession of mineral springs, can scarcely be adduced, than Leamington. Formerly an obscure hamlet, it now assumes, every day, more

and more, the pride and magnificence of a modern
town ; and promises to become highly distinguished as a watering place.   The surrounding
country is agreeable, and admirably convenient
for the invalid in the variety and facility of its
walks and rides.   Interesting objects of curiosity
in the neighbourhood are not wanting.   That ancient and most noble structure, Warwick Castle ;
the romantic attraction of Guy's Cliff; the vene-
rable ruins of Kenilworth Castle; Stratford-upon-
Avon at an accessible distance; the well-known
birth-place of our divine Shakespeare; may be
mentioned as assurances to the visitor, that in
pursuing his daily exercise he will find an ample
share of gratification.

## SPRINGS OF LEAMINGTON.

The saline springs of Leamington were noticed by many of our early writers, as by Camden,
about 1586, Speed in 1596, and by others.   Dug-
dale, in his edition of the Antiquities of Warwick-
shire, 1656, speaks of a " spring of salt water
nigh the west end of the church."

The spring, which supplied the old baths,
was discovered in the year 1786.   The new
baths were erected in 1791 ; and the spring itself
was discovered in 1790.

As the soil, which belongs to different proprietors, furnishes mineral springs in various situ-

ations, it follows, as a natural consequence of laudable enterprise, that as many pump-rooms, with all the appendages of baths, should be built. Hence the multiplication of waters, which, as may be supposed, cannot all vary in the nature of their composition. I have now to report how far the several waters, in number nine, are really distinct in character; and what is their comparative strength of impregnation.

### ROYAL PUMP ROOM.

### *Saline Water.*

The water is transparent, but not sparkling. The same observation applies to all the waters. The temperature of this and all the waters of Leamington varies with the season of the year. For example, this spring, which in November 1819 was 46°, proved, at the end of July 1820, to be 56°.

The taste of this water is strongly saline, and considerably bitter.

The specific gravity, 1·0119*.

---

* In a recent " Analysis of the Leamington Spa," &c. &c. by Dr. Weatherhead, I find the specific gravity of this water to be stated so remarkably high as 1·072. I cannot possibly account for this wide discordance with the result of my examination. I must consider this high specific gravity to be incompatible with the solid contents of the water. Dr. Amos

*Action of Tests.*

Litmus paper becomes distinctly reddened. Hyacinth paper is not affected.

To save repetition, I shall here observe, that each of the waters at Leamington gave similar evidences with these test papers, and each affected the litmus in about an equal degree; the change of colour being evanescent if allowed to dry with exposure to the open air.

Tincture of galls produces a faint purple hue; and prussiate of potash, a perceptible shade of green.

Acetate of lead, a copious white precipitate.

Solution of soap renders the water flaky.

Muriate of lime does not disturb its transparency.

Pure ammonia renders it milky.

Pure barytes causes a dense cloud.

Muriate of barytes produces a copious precipitate*.

---

Middleton makes a near approach to my number. I refer the reader to Dr. Weatherhead's Analysis, and to Dr. Middleton's printed Tabular View of the different Waters.

* As a summary mode of obtaining an estimate of the proportion of combined carbonic acid in a mineral water, Dr. Murray (Annals of Philosophy, vol. x.) gives the following formula, the free carbonic acid being removed by the previous process of concentration, which prepares it for these steps:—
" Add to the water thus concentrated a saturated solution of muriate of barytes, as long as any precipitation is produced,

Lime water renders the water milky.

Carbonate of ammonia produces a dense precipitate, and phosphate of soda added to the clear liquor, a granular precipitate.

Subcarbonate of soda, an abundant flaky precipitate.

Nitrate of silver, a copious precipitate.

Oxalate of ammonia, also a copious precipitate.

From these results we are led to conclude, that this water possesses a considerable share of

---

taking care to avoid adding an excess.    By a previous experiment, let it be ascertained whether this precipitate effervesces or not with diluted muriatic acid, and whether it is entirely dissolved.    If it is, the precipitate is of course carbonate of barytes, the weight of which, when it is dried, gives the quantity of carbonic acid ; 100 grains containing 22 of acid.    If it do not effervesce, it is sulphate of barytes, the weight of which, in like manner, gives the quantity of carbonic acid ; 100 grs. dried at a low red heat, containing 34 of acid.    If it effervesce, and is partially dissolved, it consists both of carbonate and sulphate.    To ascertain the proportion of these, let the precipitate be dried at a heat a little inferior to redness, and weighed ; then submit it to the action of dilute muriate acid ; after this wash it with water, and dry it by a similar heat, its weight will give the quantity of sulphate, and the loss of weight that of carbonate of barytes."    It was not convenient to us, with so many waters for examination, to add this step to the other numerous processes.    The carbonates, therefore, are not included in the analysis which I present of the Cheltenham and Leamington waters.    They would be inconsiderable and unimportant in the waters of Cheltenham ; and not of much amount in those of Leamington.

free carbonic acid, and that it contains lime and
magnesia, muriatic and sulphuric acids. With
respect to soda, we have no direct indication for
it by the action of re-agents ; but as it uniformly
constitutes the base with which the excess of
these acids is neutralised in all other mineral
waters, its existence may fairly be inferred here.

### Analysis.

In a pint,

Grains.

| | Grains. |
|---|---|
| Muriate of soda.......... | 53.75 |
| ———— lime.......... | 28·64 |
| ———— magnesia...... | 20·16 |
| Sulphate of soda.......... | 7:83 |
| | 110·38 |

Oxide of iron, a trace.

ROYAL PUMP ROOM.

### Sulphur Water.

The taste of this water is saline, and, together
with its odour, discovers its strong impregnation
with sulphuretted hydrogen.

Specific gravity, 1·0042.

### Action of Tests.

With respect to the saline ingredients, the
tests produced the same appearances with all the
waters, the difference being only degree, accord-

ing to the different strength of the impregnation; as will be obvious.

Acetate of lead instantly produced with this water a copious precipitate, of a deep porter colour.

Tincture of galls occasions a very faint purple hue.

Prussiate of potash, no perceptible change.

*Analysis.*

In a pint,

| | Grains. |
|---|---|
| Muriate of soda | 15·00 |
| ———— lime | 7·96 |
| ———— magnesia | 3·30 |
| Sulphate of soda | 11·60 |
| | 37·86 |

Oxide of iron, a trace.

### LORD AYLESFORD'S SPRING.

This appears to be the spring noticed by Camden. It is situated near the church, at a short distance from the Leam, and has recently been inclosed by a small but handsome structure, with a pump room.—A pump affixed to the outer part of the building is charitably allowed to the use of the poor.

The taste of this water is pleasantly saline, and slightly chalybeate.

Specific gravity, 1·0093.

Tincture of galls renders the water very slightly purple.

Prussiate of potash produces only a very slight shade of green.

Acetate of lead, a white precipitate.

### Analysis.

In a pint,

|  | Grains. |
|---|---|
| Muriate of soda | 12·25 |
| ———— lime | 28·24 |
| ———— magnesia | 5·22 |
| Sulphate of soda | 32·96 |
|  | 78·67 |

Oxide of iron, a minute portion.

### MR. ROBBINS'S SPRING.

Taste, agreeably saline.

Specific gravity, 1·0118.

Tincture of galls produces a pale purple hue.

Prussiate of potash, a shade of green, after standing, just perceptible.

Acetate of lead, a white precipitate.

### Analysis.

In a pint,

|  | Grains. |
|---|---|
| Muriate of soda | 46·75 |
| ———— lime | 17·20 |
| ———— magnesia | . . |
| Sulphate of soda | 31·20 |

Oxide of iron, a minute portion.

The quantity of muriate of magnesia cannot in the present instance be stated, from the accident of losing a portion of the precipitate. We may reasonably conjecture that its proportion would be seven or eight grains.

## MR. WISE'S SPRING.

Taste, agreeably saline.

Specific gravity, 1·010.

Tincture of galls, after some minutes, produces a very faint purple hue ; which by standing becomes a pale brown.

Prussiate of potash produces a distinct shade of green.

Acetate of lead, a white precipitate.

### *Analysis.*

In a pint,

|  | Grains. |
|---|---|
| Muriate of soda | 30·30 |
| ———— lime | 21·52 |
| ———— magnesia | 5·22 |
| Sulphate of soda | 33·44 |
|  | 90·48 |

Oxide of iron, a minute portion.

## MRS. SMITH'S SPRING.

Taste, agreeably saline, more mildly so than the other waters.

Specific gravity, 1·0085.

Tincture of galls produces a faint purple, but prussiate of potash does not occasion any perceptible change.

Acetate of lead, a white precipitate.

### *Analysis.*

In a pint,

|  | Grains. |
| --- | --- |
| Muriate of soda | 22·80 |
| ———— lime | 20·24 |
| ———— magnesia | 5·22 |
| Sulphate of soda | 28.16 |
|  | 76.42 |

Oxide of iron, a trace.

## MARBLE BATHS PUMP ROOM.

The waters are supplied to the drinkers at this pump room from urns, which are consequently the temporary reservoirs of the water. The material of these urns is cast iron, and for the use of the sulphuretted water should be exchanged for wood or stone. The water becomes blackened by the metal, from the decomposition which it undergoes with the gas; and considerable pumping is necessary before the water can be delivered clear.

*Right Urn.*—The water from this urn possesses very strongly the smell and taste of sulphuretted hydrogen. It is also strongly saline.

Specific gravity, 1·011.

Acetate of lead produces an immediate, very copious, and deep porter colour precipitate, rather darker than the sulphuretted water at the Royal Pump Room*. From a comparison also with characters written on paper with a pen dipped first in a solution of acetate of lead, and then in these waters, the permanent evidence was rather in favour of this water, as being most strongly impregnated with the gas. I do not, however, view the difference as considerable.

Tincture of galls produces a slight purple hue.

Prussiate of potash, no perceptible change.

---

* Dr. Weatherhead's results, in regard to sulphuretted hydrogen and oxide of iron, in the different waters, occasion one the greatest surprise. See his Analysis. I can only observe, with regard to my own examination, that it was made at the springs; and the experiments have since been several times repeated.

### *Analysis.*

In a pint,

|  | Grains. |
|---|---|
| Muriate of soda | 15·00 |
| ———— lime | 7·96 |
| ———— magnesia | 3·30 |
| Sulphate of soda | 11·60 |
|  | 37·86 |

Oxide of iron, a minute portion.

*Left Urn.*—The taste of the water is strongly chalybeate, and this flavour predominates over the saline.

The specific gravity, 1·0067.

Tincture of galls immediately produces a strong purple hue; which, by standing, passes into clove brown.

Prussiate of potash becomes an azure blue, which, by standing, passes into verdigris green. This water, containing a smaller proportion of saline ingredients, together with a larger proportion of oxide of iron, than the Cheltenham waters, does not modify the action of these re-agents, in regard to the shades of colour to the extent which I mentioned at p. 191. I should observe, that all the waters at Leamington containing iron cease to afford any evidence of the metal after being boiled, or being exposed for

Q

some time to the atmosphere.  Consequently the iron exists in the water, as an oxide held in solution by carbonic acid gas.

Acetate of lead produces with this water a white precipitate.

### *Analysis.*

In a pint,

|  | Grains. |
|---|---|
| Muriate of soda............... | 7·38 |
| ————— lime............ | 9·20 |
| ————— magnesia........ | 3·13 |
| ————— Sulphate of soda.. | 11.20 |

30·91

Oxide of iron, probably almost
two grains in a gallon.

*Middle Urn.*—Taste, equally saline and chalybeate.

Specific gravity 1·0054.

Tincture of galls, in about a minute, produces a lively purple; the effect much less marked than with the water from the left urn.

Prussiate of potash, in rather more time, occasions a light azure blue.

Acetate of lead produces a white precipitate.

*Analysis.*

In a pint,

Grains.

Muriate of soda............ 9·33

—————— lime.......... .... 3·07

—————— magnesia....... 6·77

Sulphate of soda.......... 8·24

_____

27·41

Oxide of iron, probably a grain
in a gallon.

From a review of the composition of all the
Leamington waters, I am led to draw the following conclusions in regard to their chemical and
medical properties. I shall endeavour to state my
opinions in the most intelligible language.

Royal Pump Room—*saline water.* This
water having only a small trace of iron, may be
considered almost as a pure saline water, strongly
alterative, and considerably aperient. It contains
so large a proportion of the muriate of lime, that
it would not, in my opinion, be proper to heighten
the power of the water by concentration ; and if
it were desired to increase the saline aperient
action, sulphate of soda or sulphate of magnesia
might be added ; but in this case, I should recommend the patient to add himself a given quan_
tity of solution of either salt. As a general rule,
I would prefer that the action of the water on the
bowels should be assisted by suitable pills taken

on the preceding night. If saline solution be
added, a pill, simply alterative, should be taken ;
but otherwise, one aperient and alterative.

Royal Pump Room—*sulphur water*.   This is
an excellent alterative water; and it is mildly
aperient.   It contains very good proportions of
the muriates of lime and magnesia, and an active
impregnation with sulphuretted hydrogen.   The
oxide of iron exists only in small proportion ;
but this will add to its efficacy as a stimulant.
Upon examining a bottle of this water several
months after I had received it in London, I found
that it had lost all trace of sulphuretted hydrogen.
It had been carefully corked and sealed at the
spring.   The Harrogate water, it will be remem-
bered (see p. 93), retains its gaseous impregnation, seemingly undiminished, for many months ;
and I am not aware of any limited time for the
continuance of this property, if the cork be carefully sealed with wax*.   The explanation of the
difference in question appears to be this. The
Leamington waters are represented, in all the analyses which have been made, to contain a portion
of atmospherical air.   If sulphuretted hydrogen be
present in a water containing atmospherical air,
we may suppose it to become converted, by keeping, into sulphuric acid, which may combine with
any basis present.   The absence of atmospherical

---

* This is much more suited to the purpose than resin.

air in the Harrogate water, and the large proportion of the gas, serve therefore to explain the
perfection in which the water may be preserved.
The change in the Leamington water takes place
slowly. I examined another bottle several weeks
after it was in my possession, and found that it
still retained, slightly, the smell and taste of the
gas, and produced a light brown precipitate with
acetate of lead. We may suppose that the water
acquires atmospherical air near the surface ; or
why should not the decomposition take place
before its arrival from the spring ?

*Lord Aylesford's Spring.* This water is considerably aperient, and very active in its alterative
properties, especially in its proportion of muriate of
lime ; which, it will be observed, exceeds the quantity contained in any of the other waters. The proportion of iron is so small, that it cannot be expected to add materially to the stimulating quality
of the water ; but if the water prove too exciting,
it may be taken after the separation of the iron ;
which, as its solvent is carbonic acid, will fall
down from simple exposure.

I wish here to correct my observation at page
19, respecting sea water, when speaking of its
large quantity of muriates of magnesia and lime.
I should rather have said, that sea water can be
taken without hazard, than without inconvenience; for, as a medicine, it is in every respect one

not delicate for the stomach, and often proves very rough in its operation. In such large doses, these muriates act directly on the bowels. In the praise which I have given to these substances, I have spoken of them as alteratives, in concurrence with the sentiments of Dr. Murray, quoted at page 141.

*Robbins's Spring.*—This water may be compared very closely to the saline at the Royal Pump Room. It contains only a minute portion of iron; and if this be thought matter of objection in any particular instance, the water may be rendered free from its chalybeate impregnation, as already explained, by simple exposure for a few hours.

*Wise's Spring.*—The same general observations are applicable to this water, as to the last. Its impregnation with sulphate of soda and muriate of lime is rather stronger; while the muriate of soda is weaker.

*Smith's Spring.*—In this water, the muriate of soda is in much smaller quantity than in the two preceding waters; the muriate of lime is very considerable; and the sulphate of soda in sufficient proportion. The oxide of iron can only be mentioned as a trace.

Marble Baths Pump Room; *Right Urn.*—This water, in its impregnation with sulphuretted hydrogen, is the nearest in strength to Harrogate

water, of all the waters which I have examined*.
In its saline contents, it is evidently altogether a
stronger water than the sulphuretted water at the
Royal Pump Room, as will appear from a comparison between the tables. In regard to the oxide
of iron, I believe the proportion to be about equal.

*Left Urn.*—This water is a very strong chalybeate alterative; and is inferior to the saline
chalybeate at Harrogate only in its proportion of
muriate of soda; while in the important muriates,
its impregnation is much stronger. I consider
it to be a water altogether of active properties.

*Middle Urn.*—This water possesses some
considerable difference of character from the preceding. In the doses in which it is taken, the
proportion of sulphate of soda becomes very
similar; the muriate of lime, a third less; the
muriate of magnesia about double; and it has
almost twice the proportion of iron.

I think it necessary, in conclusion, to offer a
few remarks on the relative qualities of the different waters, as compared with each other; and
by such additional observations I hope to give a
sufficient medical view of the subject. In my

---

* This water is, however, quite distinct from the Harrogate in its total properties. The Harrogate is still more
strongly sulphuretted, and retains the gas more intimately
combined; it is quite free from iron; and it is differently impregnated with the muriates.

report of the Harrogate and Cheltenham waters,
I have already advanced opinions which will have
a general application to these of Leamington.

The Royal Pump Room saline, is the most
pure saline water in Leamington ; that is, the most
free from chalybeate impregnation. Robbins's,
Wise's, and Smith's springs, stand in a very
equal relation to each other ; and possess so
minute a share of oxide of iron, that the waters
on that account, except in particular instances,
cannot be disapproved ; and if this be a point of
objection, either water may be freed from iron
by simple exposure, as already stated ; or the saline water at the Royal Pump Room may be
selected.

Lord Aylesford's spring differs from the last
three waters in containing a stronger impregnation with muriate of lime, and about the same
proportion of oxide of iron. Consequently, in its
medicinal action, it is to be viewed as more stimulating ; and, when increase of power is wanted,
the most worthy of preference.

The waters at the marble baths stand more
by themselves in their composition. The sulphuretted water of the right urn is stronger in its
gaseous impregnation, than the sulphur water at
the Royal Pump Room, with which it is to be compared. It contains rather more oxide of iron,
more than twice the proportion of sulphate of
soda, more than thrice of muriate of lime, and

about twice of muriate of magnesia. I would therefore pronounce that a patient should take the sulphuretted water at the Royal Pump Room first, as introductory to this the stronger. These waters will be suitable remedies in many important cases of constitutional disorders and relaxation, after the saline aperient waters have been employed for a sufficient time; or, in other instances, after an active course of aperient alterative medicines.

The water of the left urn differs from all the rest in its high degree of chalybeate power; and if we assign to the muriates their due share of influence, we must reckon this water to be highly stimulating, and as seldom fit to be employed until after a preparatory course of the pure saline water; or of medicines which have freed the habit from every material symptom of excitement and visceral obstruction.

The water of the middle urn appears to me in the same matter introductory to that of the left urn, as the one sulphuretted water is to the other, in the order just described. It is strictly so in regard to the iron which it contains, and the only question in this respect will be as respect the muriates; the most active of which it possesses in a threefold proportion. This point must be determined by the practitioner in the particular case of his patient.

The waters of Leamington, as compared with those of Cheltenham, are, according to my view of their comparative composition, considerably different in their medicinal character. The saline class are much more highly impregnated with muriate of lime; the sulphuretted in the one instance powerful, and the other almost negative; the chalybeate of very superior activity. But it does not follow that the invalid should, from this statement, give a necessary preference to the springs of Leamington. On the contrary, in all these cases in which the most saline; or, in familiar language, the most cooling aperient waters are required, Cheltenham will deserve the preference. In general terms, I am disposed to consider that the use of the waters of Cheltenham should sometimes be introductory to those of Leamington; as being less stimulating.

It would add unnecessarily, in my opinion, to the pages of this Treatise, already become too extended, if I were to pursue my medical details. The diseases which call for the use of the waters of Cheltenham, also demand the springs of Leamington; with a consideration as to the order of their employment, which must be determined by medical opinion and experience.

I wish it to be understood that all the observations which I have advanced under the head of Cheltenham Waters, as to the necessity of *fit preparation,* and combining the use of pills both alterative and aperient, are equally applicable to a course of the waters of Leamington\*.

It is but justice to add, of this watering place, which is so justly rising in public favour, that its numerous baths are constructed in a style of neatness and elegance not to be surpassed ; and the sulphuretted baths, when heated to the usual temperature, retain their gaseous impregnation in such a degree of strength, as to render them fully worthy of confidence where such a remedy is required.

---

\* Dr. Lambe published an Analysis of two of the Mineral Springs at Leamington, in the Manchester Memoirs, vol. v. part i. He describes them as the water of the New Baths, discovered in 1790 ; and water of the Old Baths, discovered in 1786. He detected the presence of manganese in each water ; but speaks of its quantity, as " unknown, but very small."

# MALVERN WELLS.

THE village of Great Malvern, distant from London 120 miles ; from the city of Worcester 8 ; and from Cheltenham 22; is situated on the east side of a chain of hills, about nine miles extending in an uninterrupted manner from north to south. " The highest of these, called the Herefordshire Beacon, is 1444 feet above the level of the sea. From the top of these hills there is a most extensive and beautiful view, but presenting on the opposite sides very different characters. Towards the west appears a succession of rising ground, terminated by the distant Welsh mountains. The eastern side of the range is the steepest, and in this direction the prospect is over the widely extended plain of Worcestershire. This side of the Malvern Hills is also much broken by narrow vallies, that run at right angles to the direction of the range. The whole of these hills is almost entirely covered with vegetation, and only in a few places, and chiefly on the eastern side, does the rock project above the surface. The rock is also generally in a state of decomposition ; and, partly from this cause, its nature is not easily ascertained. We are indebted to Leonard Horner

Esq. for a very excellent account of the mineralogy of these hills: he describes the rocks as extremely diversified in their composition, and ambiguous in their character; but as composed of felspar, hornblende, quartz, and mica, in various proportions, with, occasionally, epidote; forming unstratified rocks of the primitive class, and which may be considered as varieties of granite, sienite, and greenstone. On the western side are stratified rocks, of the transition class, chiefly the species termed graywacke, containing a few fossil shells and subordinate beds of enchrinital limestone. The dip of these rocks is various; but in general they rise towards the unstratified central mass. The plain of Worcestershire, which comes up to the bottom of the eastern side of the hills, consists of a deep alluvium covering a red sandstone, which does not occur on the western side. These hills do not give rise to any river; but throughout its whole extent, there are several small springs, some of which are found to be mineralized. Those of Malvern Wells have long been celebrated. They were first examined by Dr. Wall, of Oxford, in 1756; afterwards by Dr. W. Philip, of Worcester, in 1805."

Having premised this account of the country, with which I am obligingly favoured by Thomas Webster, Esq. the Secretary of the Geological Society, I proceed to give a brief account of the waters.

## ST. ANNE'S WELL.

This pure fountain is situated at an agreeable distance up the hill which overhangs great Malvern. The water is beautifully transparent. No crystal stream can be more clear. Received into a glass, quietly, it does not sparkle.

To the palate the water is devoid of taste; but it is highly agreeable and refreshing, and at once conveys an assurance of its purity.

I found the temperature, in September 1819, 51°.

The specific gravity, 1·0002; distilled water being considered, 1·0000.

### *Action of Tests.*

Neither litmus paper, nor that stained with the wild hyacinth, undergo any change of colour.

Nitrate of silver immediately produces a slight opalescence.

Muriate of barytes acts very slowly in disturbing the transparency of the water, and but in a slight degree.

Oxalate of ammonia acts in a similar manner.

Neither tincture of galls nor prussiate of potash produce the smallest indication of iron.

Lime water, according to Dr. Philip, does not disturb its transparency.

## Analysis.

A portion of the water was concentrated by evaporation to one-fourth, and treated in the usual manner with precipitants. A separate portion, much concentrated, gave a slight indication of magnesia, when assayed by carbonate of ammonia and phosphate of soda.

From our analysis, thus conducted, we obtained the following results.

In a gallon,

|  | Grains. |
|---|---|
| Sulphate of soda.......... | 1·940 |
| Muriate of lime.......... | 1·860 |
| Lime, ·9320, probably in union with carbonic acid, and equal to carbonate of lime....... | 1·664 |
| Magnesia, a trace........ | |

5·464

Dr. Philip, in his analysis, made in 1805, gives the following table of the composition of the water.

In a gallon,

|  | Grains. |
|---|---|
| Carbonate of soda.......... | 3·55 |
| ———— lime.......... | 0·352 |
| ———— magnesia....... | 0·26 |
| ———— iron.......... | 0·328 |
| Sulphate of soda.......... | 1·48 |
| Muriate ———— .......... | 0·955 |
| Residuum................ | 0·47 |

7·395

Dr. Saunders reports, that the Malvern water is wholly devoid of iron; and the above analysis represents the quantity to be little more than a quarter of a grain of the carbonate in a gallon\*. I could not discover, by the most careful examination, the least indication of this metal.

## THE HOLY WELL WATER.

This spring issues up the hill, midway between the villages of Great and Little Malvern. Its physical properties precisely resemble those of St. Anne's Well.

Its specific gravity is the same.

It is affected in the same manner by re-agents; and I have also to add, that our analysis furnished exactly the same results.

---

\* I feel it necessary to observe, that Dr. Philip employed, in his examination regarding the carbonate of iron, muriatic acid, prussiate of potash, and a filter not counterpoised. The muriatic acid of commerce always contains iron. It is difficult to procure it pure. The prussiate of potash is well known to contain iron. May not, therefore, the small proportion which is stated, have been derived from such sources?

At a short distance from Malvern, my attention was directed to a spring, which is well known as a chalybeate. It was much out of order at the time; but I satisfied myself that it was a simple carbonated chalybeate, and not strongly impregnated.

Dr. Philip, however, obtained double the quantity of solid contents from this water ; and in describing the action of the tests, he states thus : " To a glass of the water at the spring-head, a small quantity of lime water was added : small distinct flocculi formed, and floated throughout, but not numerous."

I am at a loss to account for these differences of result ; as, from the most careful examination, I could not discover any appreciable distinction between the two waters.

## MEDICAL HISTORY.

Dr. Saunders remarks, of Malvern, " that it has been for many years celebrated for a spring of remarkable purity, which has acquired the name of the Holy Well, from the reputed sanctity of its waters ; and the real and extensive benefit long derived in various cases from its use." He proceeds with the following account, which I believe to be abridged from the history given at length by Dr. Wall. As I have not myself had more than a slight experience of the medicinal effects of these waters, I shall present to the reader the whole quotation from Dr. Saunders' Treatise—

R

" The great benefit arising from using Malvern water as an external remedy in diseases of the skin and surface of the body, has led to its employment in some internal disorders, and often with considerable advantage. Of these, the most important are painful affections of the kidnies and bladder, attended with the discharge of bloody, purulent, or fetid urine ; the hectic fever produced by scrophulous ulceration of the lungs, or very extensive and irritating sores on the surface of the body, and also fistulas of long standing that have been neglected, and have become constant and troublesome sores.

" The Malvern water, though unquestionably of great benefit in many of the cases that we have just enumerated, is, in general, a perfectly safe application, and may be used with the utmost freedom, both as an external dressing for sores, and as a common drink ; and this is particularly the case with the common people. that resort to this spring for cutaneous complaints or other sores, who are in the constant habit of dipping their linen in the water, dressing with it quite wet, and renewing this application as often as it dries. The perfect safety of this practice on a preternaturally irritated surface, has been ascertained by long experience, and is in itself an important circumstance in illustrating the effect of moisture on the surface of the body.

" The internal use of Malvern water is sometimes attended at first with a slight nausea, and
not unfrequently, for the first day or two, it occasions some degree of drowsiness, vertigo, or
slight pain of the head, which comes on a few
minutes after drinking it. This effect Dr. Wall
ingeniously explains from the temporary plethora
of the vessels of the head, occasioned by the great
ease and rapidity with which this pure liquid
enters the absorbent system. These symptoms
go off spontaneously after a few days, or may readily be removed by a mild purgative. The effects
of this water on the bowels are not at all constant; frequently it purges briskly for a few days,
but it is not uncommon for the body to be rendered costive by its use, especially, as Dr. Wall
observes, with those who are accustomed to malt
liquors. In all cases it decidedly increases the flow
of urine, and the general health of the patient;
his appetite and spirits almost invariably improve
during a course of the water, if it agrees in the
first instance. To this, the fine mountain air,
and beauty of the situation, which tempts the invalid to active exercise, will doubtless much contribute; and the temperance and regularity of
life which is generally observed in these places
by patients of every rank, will assist in securing
the advantage which has been gained by the use
of the water.

" The duration of a course of Malvern water
must vary very considerably, on account of the
different kinds of disease for which this spring is
resorted to. Cases of obstinate scrophulous sores,
especially with caries in any bone, are always long
in healing, and require a residence here for a
considerable time. The same may be said of
very obstinate herpetic eruptions ; but where the
cutaneous affection is mild, or where a tendency
to it comes on at stated times, which is sometimes the case, this habit may be checked by a
short use of this water ; and hence some persons
who are liable to this disorder, make an annual
visit to this salubrious spring."

Of all the waters which have come under
my examination, these of Malvern claim the most
regard for their purity. I have felt it incumbent
on me to state the preceding account of the recorded virtues of these springs ; but I offer no
pledge that they possess so great an efficacy. Indeed, when we consider for a moment the remarkably slight impregnation of each water, it
becomes difficult to assign to them so large a
share of medicinal power. I am, however, most
willing to admit, that, if a course of the water,
from either spring, be united with a plan of regulated diet, both as regards the dinner meal and
the use of wine, material benefit will be derived.
I have, with success, advised the addition of

tincture of ammoniated iron to the water, in graduated doses. Any class of medicines, which a particular case may require, will be perfectly compatible with the use of the water.

This is certain.—The salubrious air of Malvern, and the peaceful feelings which the quiet and charming retirement of the spot inspires, contribute in the greatest degree to strengthen the body, to calm the mind, and thus to promote the general health. It is from such a conviction, that I have advised the Cheltenham invalid to repair to this favoured situation, at a certain period after the use of the aperient alterative waters.

If my subject permitted me to indulge in romantic description, I should find it difficult to confine my imagination when engaged in any account of Malvern; so striking are its natural beauties; so pure and restorative the air; so perfect, indeed, is the whole in every object which the mind solicits in a rural scene.

## ALUMINOUS CHALYBEATE SPRING,
### ISLE OF WIGHT.

——

AT the particular request of Mr. Waterworth, the discoverer and proprietor of this
spring, I am happy to insert a concise report of
its chemical and medicinal qualities. I have
made some examination of the specimen of the
water with which I am favoured ; but it would
not suit my present convenience to engage in its
analysis ; and, indeed, such an investigation is
rendered wholly unnecessary, from the scientific
and complete analysis* which was made by Dr.
Marcet, whose skill and philosophy in chemistry
require no praise. I shall therefore beg leave to
transcribe his details, offering such occasional
comments as the subject may suggest.

" SITUATION AND NATURAL HISTORY OF
THE SPRING.

" This spring is situated on the south-west
coast of the Isle of Wight, about two miles to

---

* Published in the Geological Transactions, vol. i.

the westward of Niton, in one of those romantic spots for which that coast is so remarkable.

" In its present state it may be said to be of difficult access, for there is no carriage road, nor even any regular foot-path along the cliff leading to it, and the walk would appear somewhat arduous to those unaccustomed to pedestrian excursions. But it would be practicable, and probably not very expensive, to render this path equally easy and agreeable    It was in walking along the shore, a few years ago, that Mr. Waterworth's attention was accidentally directed to this spring, which he traced to its present source, by observing black stains formed by rivulets flowing from that spot.

" With regard to the mineralogical history of that district, I have been favoured, through the kindness of my friend Dr. Berger, who visited the spot very lately, with so much more accurate an account of it than I should, from my own observation, have been able to offer, that I shall make no apology for transcribing it in his own words.

" The aluminous chalybeate spring," says Dr. Berger, " issues from the cliff on the S.S.W. coast of the Isle of Wight, below St. Catherine's Sea Mark, in the parish of Chale. The bearing of the needles from the spot is N.W. while that of Rockenend, not far distant, is S.E. by S.

" The elevation of the spot, as far as I could ascertain it by the barometer, is one hundred and

thirty feet above the level of the sea.   Its distance
from  the shore may 'be  about one hundred and
fifty yards.

" The water is received into a bason formed
in the rock for that purpose, and flows, as I was
informed, at the  rate of two or three hogsheads
in a day.   Its temperature I found to be 51°, that
of the atmosphere being  48° ;  and it may be
worth while to observe that this temperature cor-
responds with that of several springs of pure
water which I have met with in the island.

" The lower part of the cliff is rather in-
cumbered with masses of rock, or portions of
soil, which have fallen from the upper strata.
Immediately above these; the spring issues from
a bed of loose quartzose sandstone containing
oxyd of iron.   This sand, in which vestiges of
vegetable matter are discoverable*, alternates with
a purplish argillaceous slate of a fine grain, disposed in thin layers with a few specks of silvery
mica interspersed through the mass.   Black
stains, or impressions of vegetables, are seen on

-----

" * On being sprinkled on a heated shovel, this sand scin-
tillates as if undergoing a partial combustion.   When submitted to chemical analysis, it yields a quantity of iron, but
no lime, nor alumine, nor any other earthy matter soluble in
acid.   Close to the spring, this sand contains some traces of
sulphuric acid, but not at a distance from it: it is evident
therefore that the sand rock is not the medium through which
the spring is impregnated."

the natural joints of this rock. Above this, lies a stratum of several fathoms in thickness, of a blueish calcareous marl, with specks of mica, which has an earthy and friable texture, and contains imbedded nodules or kidneys of sulphuret of iron. Many of these nodules have undergone a partial decomposition, to which, no doubt, the existence of the principal ingredients of the spring is to be ascribed. The upper strata of the cliff are composed of a calcareous free stone, alternating with a coarse shelly limestone, accompanied by nodules or layers of *chert* or flint.

" As the same arrangement of rocks here observed prevails in several other parts of the Isle of Wight, and even along the coast of Hampshire, it is not improbable that other springs of a similar nature might be discovered. May not *Alum Bay*, which lies to the north of the Needles, have derived its name from a circumstance of this kind?

" On the road from Shorwell to Chale, the soil consists of a ferruginous sandstone, and chalybeate iridescent waters are to be seen in several places. To the east of Fresh-water Bay, not far from the place where the cliffs of chalk begin to make their appearance, there is a rivulet, the taste of which strongly indicates the presence of iron. At Blackgang Chine, a little to the N.W. of the aluminous chalybeate, is another ferruginous stream running to the sea. The rock there, is a sort of decomposed iron stone under the form of balls. The sound compact iron-stone, having the appearance of flat pebbles worn by the rolling of the sea, occurs not unfrequently along the shore."

## " GENERAL QUALITIES AND SPECIFIC GRAVITY OF THE WATER.

" *a*. The water issues from the sand rock above described, perfectly transparent, and it continues so for any length of time, provided it be collected immediately, and preserved in perfectly closed vessels ; but if allowed to remain in contact with the air, or even if corked up after a temporary exposure to it, reddish flakes are soon deposited, which partly subside, and partly adhere to the inside of the vessel.

" *b*. It has no smell, except that which is common to all chalybeates, and this it possesses but in a very slight degree.

" *c*. Its taste is intensely chalybeate\*, and, besides a considerable degree of astringency and harshness, it has the peculiar kind of sweetness which sulphate of iron and sulphate of alumine are known to possess.

---

\* I find the harsh astringency of the alum to be so powerfully predominant, as almost to conceal the chalybeate taste.

" *d.* Its specific gravity somewhat varies in different specimens. In three different trials I obtained the following results:

| | |
|---|---|
| 1st specimen............ | 1008·3 |
| 2nd specimen............ | 1007·2 |
| 3d specimen............. | 1006·9 |
| | 3022·4 |
| which gives a mean specific gravity of............. | 1007·5 |

" PRELIMINARY EXPERIMENTS ON THE
EFFECTS OF RE-AGENTS.

" A. Paper stained with litmus was distinctly reddened by the water.

" B. Paper stained with Brazil-wood was changed to a deep purple.

" C. When agitated in contact with the air, or repeatedly poured from one vessel into another, the water became turbid, and, on standing, deposited reddish flakes.

" D. On applying heat to a portion of the water just uncorked, and boiling it *quickly*, till it was reduced to one-half or even one-third of its original bulk, no precipitation whatever took place; but on continuing the evaporation, a white feathery crystalline substance appeared on the surface of the fluid, and on pushing the process still further, a saline matter of a pale yellowish green colour appeared, which continued to increase till the whole was reduced to a dry yellowish mass. These were the phenomena observed with water recently uncorked; but when, previous to the evaporation, it had been for some time exposed to the air, or when the evaporation was conducted very slowly, an appearance of reddish flakes was the first circumstance observed.

" E. The mineral acids produced no obvious change in the water.

" F. Oxalic acid produced a slight yellowish tinge; but no immediate precipitation or turbidness.

" G. Oxalate of ammonia, in small quantity, likewise produced a yellow colour, without precipitate: but on adding more of this test a white precipitate appeared.

" H. Prussiate of potash and infusion of galls produced abundant precipitates, the one blue, and the other black or dark purple; and the colour of these precipitates· was much paler when the water had not previously been exposed to the atmosphere.

" I. Alkaline solutions produced copious greenish flocculent precipitates, which became darker on standing in the air.

" K. Nitrate of silver occasioned a dense, white, but not considerable, precipitate.

" L. Both muriate and nitrate of barytes occasioned copious white precipitates.

" M. A piece of marble being boiled for some time in a few ounces of the water, the marble was found to have undergone no sensible loss of weight by that operation; but its surface had required a faint yellowish tinge.

" N. A quantity of the water being evaporated to dryness, and a considerable degree of heat applied to the dry residue, a solution of this in water had the same effect of reddening litmus as before.

" INFERENCES ARISING FROM THOSE EFFECTS.

" 1. From experiment A, connected with experiments C, H, I, M, and N, and from the circumstance of taste, and other general properties, it appeared highly probable that the water contained sulphate of iron, and perhaps also sulphate of alumine, without any uncombined acid*.

" 2. From experiments C and D, it appeared evident that iron and lime were contained in the water, and that their solvent was not carbonic acid†.

---

" * Solutions of sulphate of iron and sulphate of alumine, though made from these salts in their crystallized state, have, like acids, the power of imparting a red colour to litmus.

" † The reddish flakes mentioned in C and D, and in § ii, a, are uniformly found to be sub-sulphate of iron.

" The experiments D and E, concurred to show that the water did not contain any sensible quantity of carbonates.

" 4. The experiments F and G afforded additional evidence of the presence of iron, and whilst they shewed the existence of lime in the water, seemed to indicate that the quantity of this earth was not considerable.

" 5. It appeared probable from experiment K, that the water contained a small quantity of muriatic acid.

" 6. The change produced in experiment B, on the infusion of Brazil-wood, appeared at first ambiguous; it could not be owing to the prevalence of an alkali or carbonated earth, since the water turned litmus red, and since the presence of carbonated earths had been disproved by other results.   But having found, by comparative trials, that solutions of sulphate of iron changed paper stained with infusions of Brazil-wood to a black, or at least intensely dark violet colour, and that solutions of alum turned it crimson ; and observing that a mixture of these solutions produced a dark purple hue, the appearance in question was easily explained.

" 7. The result of experiment L indicated the presence of sulphuric acid.

" 8 Upon the whole, and from a review of the foregoing experiments, the substance which at this early state of the analysis, the waters appeared most likely to contain, were, *sulphate of iron, sulphate of alumine, sulphate of lime,* and a small quantity of *muriatic salts.* Some sulphate of magnesia, and some alkaline sulphates, might possibly be contained in the water, though their presence could not be satisfactorily ascertained by these preliminary experiments."

For the sake of convenient brevity, I shall refrain from quoting any part of the analytical details, and state only the final results ; referring the reader to the original paper, from which he will derive equal amusement and instruction.

" On reviewing and connecting together all the foregoing results, it appears that each pint, or sixteen-ounce measure, of the aluminous chalybeate, contains the following ingredients :

" Of carbonic acid gas three-tenth of a cubic. inch.

Grains.

Sulphate of iron, in the state of crystallized green sulphate...................................................... 41·4

Sulphate of alumine, a quantity which, if brought to the state of crystallized alum, would amount to . 31·6

Sulphate of lime, dried at 160°...................... .. 10·1

Sulphate of magnesia, or Epsom salt, crystallized... 3·6

Sulphate of soda, or Glauber salt, crystallized...... 16·0

Muriat of soda, or common salt, crystallized......... 4·0

Silica................................ ...................................... 0·7

107·4

" I am not acquainted with any chalybeate or aluminous spring, in the chemical history of mineral waters, which can be compared, in regard to strength, with that just described. The Hartfell water, and that of the Horley-green spa near Halifax, both of which appear to be analogous to to this in their chemical composition, and were considered as the strongest impregnations of the kind, are stated by Dr. Garnett to contain, the one only about 14 grs. and the other 40 grs. of saline matter in each pint.

" No doubt therefore can be entertained that the water which is the subject of this essay, will be found to possess in a very eminent degree the medical properties which are known to belong to the saline substances it contains. Indeed there appears to be in that spring rather a redundance than a deficiency of power, and it is probable that in many instances it will be found expedient to drink the water in a diluted state; whilst in others, when it may be desirable to take in a small compass large doses of these saline substances, it will be preferred in its native undiminished strength."

It is difficult, from the low state of exsiccation of the salts, to adapt the above according to Dr. Murray's view. We have considered that sulphate of lime dried at 160° may retain half its water. On this supposition, and upon the idea that the corresponding sulphate of soda contains water in a similar proportion, the following will be nearly the estimate.

In a pint,

| | Grains. |
|---|---|
| Sulphate of iron | 41·4 |
| ———— alumina | 31·6 |
| ———— lime | 7·2 |
| Muriate of lime | 2·16 |
| ——— magnesia | 1·38 |
| Sulphate of soda | 22·96 |
| Silica | 70 |
| | 107·4 |

The muriatic acid may also be supposed to be partly in combination with the alumina and iron. In consequence of all the salts having been computed in the state of crystallization, an erroneous idea is conveyed of the strength of the impregnation of this water. If all the salts were perfectly dry, the weight of the solid contents would be reduced to almost half. For example, 100 parts of crystallized sulphate of soda contain only 44 of real sulphate. 100 parts of crystallized sulphate of iron contain of dry sulphate 55 parts; and the same quantity (100 parts) would represent nearly one fourth of oxide of iron. Alum contains so large a proportion of

s

water of crystallization, that, in becoming dry, it
loses nearly half its weight.

This view of the analysis appears to me important on medical grounds; for although it is
unquestionably a water of great medicinal power,
the tabular statement which Dr. Marcet has given,
may possibly convey a mistaken notion of its
strength to the professional reader.

## MEDICAL HISTORY.

THE composition of this water clearly points
out the leading character of its nature as a medicine.  Next to the muriate of iron, the sulphate
is the strongest of the salts of iron which we possess; and the usual range of doses which we
prescribe, is from one to six grains.  The sulphate of alum is an active astringent, and hence
we have already two ingredients of considerable
power.  If we suppose that the water contains
some portion of muriate of iron and muriate of
alum, our estimate of its strength is still increased.
The muriate of lime is in efficacious quantity;
and the muriate of magnesia is in sufficient proportion to produce an alterative effect.  The sulphate of soda will tend to prevent the restringent
action of the water on the bowels.  It is evidently

in chronic diseases of relaxation, when no inflammatory action is present, that the medicinal
employment of this water is pointed out. Its
strongly styptic taste seems of itself to dictate the
necessity of commencing its use in a state of dilution ; and the degree of this dilution must be
proportioned to the delicacy of the stomach, in
every particular case.

I conceive, however, that in this division of my
subject, I cannot do so much justice to the character of the spring, as by quoting some pages
from the able and candid report of the medicinal
properties of this water, published by Dr. Lempriere, who had the opportunity with the sick
under his care at the Depôt in the Isle of Wight,
of administering the water upon an extensive
scale.

This Physician gives a tabular view of the
diseases which preceded a course of the mineral
water, with the result. The following is the list.
Continued fever, 17; agues, 90 ; pulmonic diseases, 18 ; chronic dysentery, 8 ; chronic rheumatism with emaciation, 27 ; diseases of the ab-
dominal viscera, including cases of anasarca, 21 ;
asthenia, 10. The number benefited was 140 ;
and 24 patients were taking the water: 27 had
omitted it.

In describing the operation of the water, Dr.
Lempriere proceeds with the following statement;
which, as it serves to convey a clear account of

s 2

the remedy, I shall take the liberty of presenting without abridgment.

" In giving this water, I was very forcibly struck with the rapid effect it produced on the appetite and spirits, and the confidence it inspired in the mind of the patient. In the course of a few days, from the urgent solicitations of the sick, it was found necessary to add to their ordinary allowance of animal food and vegetables *, a quarter of a pound of meat and half a pound of potatoes ; and, with a view to recovery, each was ordered one pint of porter per diem.

" The improvement of the appetite was soon succeeded by an increase of strength and a return of the natural complexion ; and the recovery of these patients evidently proved more permanent, than that of any of the other Walcheren cases sent out of hospital under a different mode of treatment.

" The water did not appear to produce any immediate effect on the pulse, or skin, nor did it act particularly on the kidnies ; its tendency to increase the appetite, and raise the spirits, was the only evident effect to be observed during the early course ; and a return of strength and general appearance of improved health, marked its latter progress.

---

" * The allowance above alluded to, consisted of half a pound of beef, or mutton, one pound of bread, and three quarters of a pound of potatoes, per diem."

" In administering the water, it was a rule, previously to devote one day to clearing the bowels by a suitable aperient ; and the sulphate of magnesia, or Epsom salts, was the medicine generally preferred.  Under this preparation, the water seldom produced any disagreeable effect on the stomach or bowels, or rendered it necessary, during the course, to take laxative medicines ; an advantage which does not attach to the other chalybeate waters, unless they hold in solution a considerable portion of some aperient salt.

" From the active substances contained in the aluminous chalybeate water, Dr. Saunders, as well as Dr. Marcet, have very judiciously recommended, that, in the first instance, it be diluted.  To patients with delicate stomachs, or in irritable habits, this precaution, as well as that of taking off the chill by immersing the glass in warm water, seems adviseable ; but in the Walcheren cases, the only qualification the water received, was the addition of a drachm, or teaspoonful of the compound tincture of cardamoms, to each dose, which at first was only two ounces, or a small wine glass full ; and this was repeated three times a day, giving the water at those periods which would the least interfere with the hours of meal.  When first prescribed, it was thought adviseable that it should not be taken in the morning fasting ; but in this, as well as in many other particulars, the practitioner must act, as circum-

stances shall suggest, bearing in recollection, that
tonic medicines, in general, produce the greatest
effect upon an empty stomach.

" In about three days, the dose of the water
was increased to three ounces, or a larger wine
glass full, with the same proportion of tincture of
cardamoms, three times a day ; and at intervals,
it was thus gradually augmented, until a pint, in
four doses, could be taken in the twenty-four
hours, though, in most instances, twelve ounces,
or three quarters of a pint, were found sufficient.

" The water, no doubt, might occasionally be
given without the tincture of cardamoms or any
other addition ; but independently of the risk
which would thereby be incurred, of nauseating
the stomach, it seems to have derived considerable efficacy from being combined with an aromatic ; in the choice of which, the practitioner
must be regulated by the habits and constitution
of the patient, as well as by the particular case
thus brought under his consideration.

" In a course of this water, costiveness, which,
with me, the remedy seldom induced, is *most
particularly* to be guarded against, by the occasional use of a suitable aperient, of which the sulphate of magnesia, or the aloetic pill with myrrh,
was generally preferred ; and a laxity of the
bowels, if it extends beyond a *temporary* effect,
may easily be restrained by adding to each dose
a few drops of the tincture of opium, or, if further

necessary, by qualifying it with some aromatic astringent.

" As the water had hitherto proved so beneficial, and as, in the first instance, it was an object to ascertain its efficacy, uninfluenced by the aid of any other remedy ; I seldom was induced to vary the mode of giving it in the cases which have been the subject of the present report ; but as the aluminous chalybeate is not liable, like most of the other mineral waters, to rapid decomposition, I am convinced it might advantageously be used in extemporaneous prescription ; so as to blend with it, either by admixture, or by a separate preparation, various other articles of the materia medica, that might not only give efficacy to the water itself, but also conjointly promote the cure, in instances, where each remedy, by itself, might possibly fail.

" Thus, in obstinate agues, as also in many other complaints where debility forms a leading feature, the water, qualified with suitable aromatics, might serve as a vehicle for the Peruvian bark, or for any of the vegetable tonics ; in chlorosis, it might to advantage be conjoined with aloes, myrrh, and one of the bitter extracts put together in the form of pills ; and in cases of anasarca, good effects might be expected, from a combination of this water with a course of diuretics, of which, perhaps, in such cases, pills composed of one of the mercurial preparations, squills, and a suitable aromatic, may be considered the best. From this view of the subject I have very lately commenced a trial of the mineral water with other remedies, the result of which may perhaps be the subject of a future communication.

" Under all circumstances, it would seem adviseable to begin the water in very small proportions ; and where, from the nature of the complaint, or from the peculiarity of the constitution of the patient, there appears to be the least risk of nauseating, it should uniformly be taken in a very diluted state, and this should not be altered, nor the proportion be increased, until the practitioner is well assured it may be done, not only with safety, but with increased advantage to the patient."

The author adds the following judicious observations :

" A nutritive diet without excess; a rigid attention to the state of the bowels, so as to avoid costiveness ; early hours, particularly early rising ; exercise in the open air, more especially on horseback ; and sea bathing, when not otherwise forbid, are among the useful auxiliaries to a course of this water ; and as probably most of the cases in which the water will be recommended, have been of long standing, and are of an obstinate nature, the patient must not be too sanguine in expecting an early cure, or fail to persevere in its use, so long as his medical adviser shall deem it requisite."

It is a pleasing consideration, that the virtues of this aluminous chalybeate spring will be materially promoted by the salutary influence of the air, and the agreeable inducements to the patient to take daily exercise, which, this beautiful island, distinguished by the exalted appellation of the *Garden of England*, every where offers.

I now conclude my Chemical and Medical Report ; and shall feel amply rewarded for my labours, if I have succeeded in exhibiting a faithful view of my subject, in some measure corresponding with its interest and importance.

FINIS.

J. Mallett, Printer, No 59, Waidour Street, Soho, London.

9 781108 062022